Rapid Review

for the

Plastic Surgery

In-Service & Board

Examinations

L. Vaughn, M.D.

This book is not intended for clinical use, and the application of information contained herein is the sole responsibility of the practitioner. The author and publishers are not liable for errors or omissions of the book or any consequences of its application. We make no expressed or implied warranty with respect to the completeness or accuracy contained in the book. Information contained in this book was obtained from a review of the ASPS In-Service examination, current textbooks, publications, and board study guides. The ASPS and the American Board of Plastic Surgery, Inc. do not sponsor or endorse this book.

This book was designed to streamline preparation for the plastic surgery in-service and board examinations. Over ten years of published in-service examination questions were reviewed and topics were organized into a concise format. This high-yield review will assist in rapid recall of information and is easier to navigate than reviewing old examinations with lengthy explanations. All of the most common topics tested are represented. More detailed information should be sought in appropriate textbooks.

Good luck!

L. Vaughn, M.D.

Contents

1. Anesthesia / Local Anesthetics

- PABA local anesthetics (esters- chloroprocaine, tetracaine, procaine & benzocaine) cause most allergic reactions. Amide local anesthetics do not metabolize to PABA so hypersensitivity is rare
- Protein binding results in ↑ DOA- ↑bupivacaine vs. lidocaine
- Lipid solubility of local anesthetic determines potency. ↑ solubility = ↑ potency
- Bupivacaine has longer onset of action (5-8 min) than lidocaine (2-4 min), but its DOA (10 hrs) is longer than lidocaine (3 hrs)
- Max dose lidocaine with 1:100,000 epinephrine- 7 mg/kg. In a 50-kg patient, the max dose is 350 mg. 1% lidocaine with 1:100,000 epinephrine contains 10 mg/1mL. Max dose is 35mL.
- Lidocaine up to 35 mg/kg is safe when given as tumescent with epinephrine
- Max dose bupivacaine is 2.5 mg/kg. 0.5% solution contains 5 mg/ml. Overdose- irreversible heart block. Rx- intralipid
- Lidocaine toxicity- initial signs- anxiety, tinnitus & perioral numbness. Later- muscle twitching, seizures, respiratory & circulatory arrest. Rx- airway, O_2, IVF. RF- obesity, HTN, Bier block
- At toxic levels lidocaine & bupivacaine block Na channels in cardiac tissue, ↓ depolarization, ↑ QRS width, ↓ L ventricular function & ventricular arrhythmias
- Epinephrine ↑ lidocaine safety by slowing absorption, allowing ↓ dose. ↑ duration of lidocaine provides longer pain relief. Vaso-constriction ↓ bleeding & OR time. Epinephrine can be used in fingers & toes
- Max amount epinephrine 1:200,000 given to child is 30mL (3 mL/kg) every 10 min
- Epinephrine extravasation Rx- elevate extremity. Phentolamine (α-blocker) may worsen injury due to pressure necrosis. Warm or cold compresses may worsen tissue damage
- Infiltrated chemo Rx- saline flush-out using stab incisions, elevate the extremity
- Absorption of tumescent lidocaine from above clavicles peaks @ 5 hrs, trunk @ 12 hrs
- Tumescent lidocaine- 0.05% solution with epinephrine 1:1,000,000. Very slow rate of absorption from subcutaneous tissue, which prevents toxicity. 1% solution max plasma concentration @ 1 hour, tumescent solution @ 8 to 12 hours
- Bier block used for short procedures on upper extremities. Tourniquet use is contraindicated in Raynaud, sickle cell, severe HTN, uncooperative or young patients
- Ketamine- IV is safe with a lower rate of laryngospasm, shorter DOA & ↓vomiting. Titrate with a continuous infusion or repeat boluses
- Malignant hyperthermia- AD. Fatal reaction to anesthetics & depolarizing neuromuscular blocking agents. MC- isoflurane & succinylcholine. S/S- muscle rigidity, tachycardia, fever, arrhythmias, metabolic & respiratory acidosis, hypotension. Early sign- tachycardia, ↑ CO_2. Late sign- hyperthermia. Rx- dantrolene

end tidal
CO_2

5

- Methemoglobinemia- Hg cannot carry O_2 to organs due to methemoglobin. Dark, reddish-brown blood. Rx- O_2, remove offending agent, antidote methylene blue. MC- topical benzocaine

  treat hyperkalemia
- Succinylcholine-induced hyperkalemia- large burns, long hospitalizations. May cause fatal cardiac arrhythmias. ↑ acetylcholine receptors. Rx- supportive measures, calcium, glucose, insulin, albuterol, lasix, kayexalate
- Post-op N/V- female, history of motion sickness, non-smoker, use of post-op opioids. Propofol prevents this. Occurs in 25-30% of surgeries. Rx- scopolamine, Zofran, steroids. ↑ local anesthetic use ↓ narcotics & N/V
- Scopolamine- centrally-acting anticholinergic agent patch placed behind ear that delivers 1.5 mg of scopolamine transdermally over 3 days. SE- sedation, dry mouth, blurred vision, mydriasis
- EMLA- topical anesthesia. Combination lidocaine & prilocaine. Absorption varies with skin thickness & vascularity. Cover with tegaderm for 1 hr
- Cocaine- max dose is 1.5 mg/kg
- Diazepam & benzodiazepines- pregnancy class D
- Bupivacaine, morphine & fentanyl- pregnancy class B/C

2. Liposuction

- Dry technique (no additional infiltrate), wet technique (200-300 mL per site), super-wet technique (1:1 ratio), or tumescent technique (3:1 ratio)
- Use epinephrine in wetting solution for vasoconstriction
- ↓ risk of lidocaine toxicity in large-volume liposuction cases by ↓ concentration of lidocaine or ↓volume of infiltrate
- 70% of infiltrate remains in patient's body. Fluid requirements = maintenance fluid + aspirate removed + fluid infiltrated

  also medial antebrachial cutaneous N.
- Suction lipoplasty of upper arm- avoid medial portion around bicipital groove where fat layer is very thin to prevent wrinkling
- Ultrasound-assisted lipoplasty- ultrasound energy disrupts fat cell. Liquefied fat is aspirated. Prevent thermal injuries to skin by infiltrating tumescent, keep probe in constant motion. ↑ seromas, tissue damage, neuropraxia
- MC complication- contour irregularity 20%. DVT <1%. Cutaneous hyperpigmentation 4%. Seromas & wound infections are rare
- MC deformity- surface irregularity due to large cannula, single port, superficial suctioning
- Mesotherapy- subcutaneous injection of medications as a nonsurgical alternative to suction lipectomy. Not good & not approved by FDA
- Large-volume liposuction- >5 L of lipoaspirate taken in one operation
- Liposuction alone worsens skin laxity by disrupting musculocutaneous suspensory fascia
- Lipobrachioplasty- combines liposuction & excision

6

- Zones of adherence- where superficial fascial system attaches to fascia of underlying muscles. Example- lateral gluteal depression superior, lateral thigh
- Fat embolism syndrome- liposuction risk. S/S- respiratory distress, ↓ cerebral function, petechial rash. Occurs within 48hrs post-op. Microparticles of fat shower lung, brain, kidney, skin. Mortality= 15%
- Fat necrosis- devascularization of fatty tissue

3. Brachioplasty

- Medial antebrachial cutaneous nerve- superficial to deep fascia, travels with basilic vein. Injury- numbness & pain near elbow. Avoid by leaving 1cm of tissue over deep fascia
- Wound dehiscence risk when liposuction is performed with brachioplasty
- Hypertrophic scarring- 40% incidence
- Anchor brachioplasty- anchors soft tissues of posteromedial aspect of arm to axillary fascia. Prevents relaxation of axillary fascia sling
- Limited incision brachioplasty- ellipse in the axilla +/- liposuction
- Traditional brachioplasty- T-shaped scar along arm & axilla

4. Lower Body Lift

- Indicated for patients with buttock & thigh ptosis
- Femoral triangle- inguinal ligament, adductor longus muscle, sartorius muscle. Iliopsoas muscle, pectineus muscle, inguinal lymph nodes, great saphenous vein & femoral nerve, artery & vein are within the femoral triangle
- Colles fascia- deep layer of superficial perineal fascia. Anteriorly continuous with Scarpa's fascia of the abdominal wall
- Lateral femoral cutaneous nerve- anterolateral thigh burning or numbness, worse with standing, walking, hip extension
- Genitofemoral nerve- proximal thigh @ femoral triangle. SE of hernia repair
- Iliohypogastric nerve- small area superior to pubis
- Ilioinguinal nerve- pubic symphysis, superomedial aspect of femoral triangle, anterior scrotum or mons pubis & labia majora
- Saphenous nerve- thigh & knee pain, paresthesias of leg & foot
- Autologous gluteal augmentation flaps- vascularized by superior & inferior gluteal arteries, can be used during lower body lifts to add volume & projection to buttocks
- Fascial anchoring technique for medial crescentic thigh lift- inferior thigh flap is anchored to fascia with subdermal sutures to reduce scar migration, labial spreading & thigh ptosis
- Medial thigh lift incision is superficial through fat over femoral triangle to preserve lymphatics

7

- Severe medial thigh skin redundancy after weight loss- medial longitudinal approach removes the most skin along entire thigh
- MC complication- seroma 37%, wound dehiscence 12%, infection 8%, PE 6%
- Body lift early wound dehiscence due to patient movement. Late wound dehiscence due to seroma

5. Abdominoplasty

- Traditional abdominoplasty- mobilization of abdominal pannus, addresses laxity above & below navel, incorporates progressive tension sutures
- Fleur-de-Lis abdominoplasty- vertical incision
- Panniculectomy- excise pannus without undermining to ↓ risk of wound complications, especially in smokers
- Thermage- not effective for lax skin
- Incision placed 5-7cm above vulvar commissure within hair. Excess mons fat treated with liposuction or excision
- Miniabdominoplasty does not address supraumbilical skin redundancy
- Neuropathic pain after abdominoplasty- injury to lateral femoral cutaneous, iliohypogastric or ilioinguinal nerve. Rx- nerve block of trigger point. Steroid block may give long-term relief. Exploration, neurectomy, replantation may be indicated
- MC nerve injured- lateral femoral cutaneous nerve. S/S- anterior, lateral thigh burning, tingling, numbness that ↑ with standing, walking
- Ilioinguinal nerve injury- inguinal paresthesia or groin, labia, scrotum, inner thigh pain
- Abdominal wall blood supply- intercostal arteries, superior & inferior superficial epigastric arteries, perforators of deep superior epigastric arteries
- Abdominoplasty divides superficial inferior epigastric arteries & perforators from rectus muscles. Flap survives on intercostal vessels. Subcostal scar is problem
- Highest risk procedure of post-op mortality from PE
- TAP regional block- thoracolumbar nerves that innervate anterior abdominal wall travel between the internal oblique & transverse abdominis muscles
- Seroma- MC complication. Dx- ballottable swelling, fluid wave. Rx-needle aspiration. If prolonged, may require operative excision. RF-obesity, concomitant liposuction, large skin resections, shear forces. Compression garments do not prevent seromas
- Rectus muscle diastasis- men upper, women lower
- Can be combined with any approach for hysterectomy
- Adding liposuction ↑ risk of skin necrosis in Zone I of abdomen

6. Breast

Medial pectoral nerve - pec major, pec minor

- Nipple innervation- 4th intercostal nerve
- Lateral pectoral nerve- pectoralis major muscle
- Long thoracic nerve- serratus anterior muscle
- Supraclavicular nerve- skin of the upper breast
- Thoracodorsal nerve- latissimus dorsi muscle
- Thoracoacromial artery & vein deep to pec major supply overlying breast tissue & skin Subglandular augmentation disrupts this, leads to possible wound-healing problems. Submuscular augmentation maintains this, allows better healing
- Nipple-to-IMF dimension ↑ over time
- Anterior thoracic hypoplasia- anterior chest wall depression resulting from posteriorly displaced ribs, breast hypoplasia, superiorly displaced NAC. Sternum & pec major are normal
- Pectus excavatum- MC congenital chest wall abnormality. Ribs & sternum form abnormally resulting in concave chest wall
- Pectus carinatum- sternum & ribs are forced anteriorly, pigeon chest
- Poland syndrome- subclavian artery supply disrupted during 6th week of gestation. Unilateral congenital anomaly. Absence of sternal head of pec major, hypoplasia of breast/nipple, ↓subcutaneous fat & axillary hair, abnormal rib cage, upper extremity.
- Sternal cleft- rare congenital defect. Failure of midline fusion of sternum, lack of protection of heart/great vessels
- Axillary accessory breast tissue- remove surgically. S/S- asymptomatic, pain, ↓ arm movement, cosmesis
- Tubular breast deformity- constricted base, high IMF, herniating nipple/areola. SE of augmentation- double bubble. Rx- breast augmentation with radial scoring & areola reduction
- Polymastia- accessory or ectopic. Ectopic breast tissue- outside the milk line (MC- dorsal thigh). Accessory polymastia- along the milk line (axilla, groin, vulva, medial thigh)
- Polythelia- increased risk of other anomalies. Needs physical exam, UA, & renal US
- Amazia- absence of glandular tissue, due to surgical removal of the breast bud, XRT, or congenital absence
- Athelia- absence of the nipple
- Jejune syndrome- narrow thorax, polychondrodystrophy, renal disease
- Amastia- absence of both breast & nipple
- Nipple inversion- failure of mammary pit to elevate above skin
- Phyllodes tumor- benign, large fibroadenoma. Rx- excise with 1cm margins, annual surveillance. May recur
- Giant fibroadenoma- solitary, firm, nontender, rapid enlargement, overlying veins, ulceration, >5cm, occur at puberty. Rx- enucleation, breast reduction
- Juvenile breast hypertrophy- unilateral or bilateral, enlargement without mass, occurs at puberty, doesn't regress, caused by estrogen stimulation. Rx- breast reduction

↑ response to estrogen by end organ, normal receptor density

- Benign premature thelarche- breasts develop before puberty. Rx- monitor
- McCune-Albright syndrome- polyostotic fibrous dysplasia- premature puberty, menses before breasts, bone abnormalities, gigantism, café spots
- Burn patient with growing breasts- Integra allows expansion, cover with STSG

7. Breast Augmentation

- Saline breast prosthesis
    - Rupture is easier to detect
- Silicone breast prostheses
    - No delay in detection of breast cancer
    - Less likely to show superior pole rippling
    - No association with connective tissue diseases
    - Must be 22 years old
    - No ↑ silicone levels in breast milk
    - 3rd generation implant- inner barrier on elastomer shell ↓ silicone bleeding
- Max prosthesis size determined by breast base width
- ↑ prosthesis volume with ↓ skin envelope results in ↓ NAC sensation
- Transaxillary augmentation- subdermal dissection, avoiding axillary fat which has branches of intercostobrachial & medial brachial cutaneous nerves (provide sensation to medial arm)
- Soft-tissue thickness <2 cm on upper pole of breast will increase the chance of rippling & wrinkling with subglandular placement
- Rippling occurs with textured & saline implants
- Augmented women get mammogram with Eklund views- implant pushed back against chest wall
- MRI of silicone implants- highest sensitivity & specificity for detecting rupture. Screening- 3 years post-op, then every 2 years thereafter. S/S- hard knots, change in size or shape, pain, tingling, swelling, numbness, burning, hardening
- Linguine sign- intracapsular silicone prosthesis rupture. Shell floating in gel
- Double-bubble deformity- native glandular tissue drops to lower pole of an implant or an implant falls below IMF
- Double capsule phenomenon- capsule over implant & another lining pocket. S/S- late-onset swelling without infection. Subglandular = submuscular
- Infected implant Rx- remove implant, irrigation, debridement, reinsertion 6 months later
- Capsular contracture- ↓ with submuscular placement, texturing. MC in first 2 years after subglandular implants. Possibly due to infection, silicone gel diffusion, smoking. Incidence- 5% @ 1 year, 18% @ 3 years

10

- Recurrent contracture- implant removal, capsulectomy, autologous flap reconstruction
- Baker Classification of Capsular Contracture After Breast Augmentation
    Class I- Normal breast; augmentation not noticeable
    Class II- Minimal contracture; implant palpable but not visible
    Class III- Moderate contracture; implant is palpable, visible
    Class IV- Severe contracture; breast is distorted, hard, cool, painful
- Synmastia- breast prosthesis crosses midline. MC- large prostheses, large base diameter, multiple surgeries, preexisting chest wall abnormality, subpectoral positioning of prostheses
- Atypical nontuberculous mycobacterium- occurs in presence of foreign bodies (breast prostheses). S/S- erythema, swelling, clear drainage. Dx- acid-fast bacilli staining & mycobacterial cultures. Rx- remove prosthesis, debride, 6 months cipro & bactrim. Replace implant after 6 months
- ALCL- extremely rare. Occurs in capsule. No evidence that breast prostheses cause ALCL. S/S- late-onset, persistent seroma, pain, lumps, swelling, asymmetry. Dx- US-guided needle aspiration
- Dissatisfaction with breast size after initial implantation leads to reoperation- thinning of tissue, shrinkage, sagging, palpable implant, visible implant, rippling and sensory loss. Shrinkage of breast tissue occurs with all prostheses; ↑prosthesis, ↑shrinkage
- Aug revision- size or shape change (30%), leakage or deflation (20%), contracture (18%), wrinkling (5%), infection (5%)

TB myiobachwn → 6 mith TB truk

8. Mastopexy

- Mastopexy blood supply
    o Superior- IMA 2nd interspace
    o Inferior/central- IMA 4th interspace
    o Medial- 3rd superficial branch of IMA
    o Lateral- lateral thoracic
- Grade 1- mild ptosis- nipple within 1cm of IMF. Rx-subglandular augmentation or circumareolar mastopexy
- Grade 2- moderate ptosis- nipple is 1-3 cm below IMF. Rx- vertical mastopexy
- Grade 3- severe ptosis- nipple >3cm below IMF, medial NAC, lateral breast mound, axillary fat roll, lower IMF, glandular tissue loss, deflated. Rx- Wise mastopexy
- Pseudoptosis (bottoming out)- breast gland migrates lower than IMF, nipple in normal position
- Augmentation mammaplasty & mastopexy- ↑ prosthesis size = ↓vascularity. NAC & skin flap loss, infection, exposure, deformities, tissue thinning, rippling, ptosis
- Vertical mammoplasty- central vertical glandular excision narrows breast, uses adjustable markings, upper pedicle, ↓undermining of the

11

skin, less scars. Contraindications- length of pedicle, amount & quality of skin
- Secondary mastopexy SE- ptosis, tissue stretching & thinning, inadequate soft-tissue coverage. Inferior pedicle is unreliable
- ↑ ptosis = ↑ reoperation rate

Superior medial most reliable

9. Gynecomastia

- Causes- amphetamines, cimetidine, digitalis, haloperidol, isoniazid, methyldopa, opiates, progestins, spironolactone, tricyclic antidepressants, ↑ estrogen (testicular tumor), ↓estrogen (klinefelters, orchiectomy)
- Wait 12 months before gynecomastia surgery. Do not order labs if no other clinical history or physical findings. If ↑ β-hCG, US testes to rule out tumor
- Lipectomy done in deeper subcutaneous plane & transitions to subdermal plane for greater skin retraction. Disruption of IMF allows more natural skin draping
- Severe gynecomastia reconstruction- position of the new NAC is oval, placed at 4th-5th intercostal space
- Pseudogynecomastia- aka lipomastia. Rx- reduction mammaplasty with repositioning of nipple, areola reduction, removal of excess skin and fat. Not proven Rx- RFA, phosphatidylcholine, liposuction does not address excess skin or large areolae
- 1% malignancy in adolescents undergoing subcutaneous mastectomy for gynecomastia

10. Breast Reconstruction

- ACS recommends annual mammogram starting at age 40
- MRI screening recommendations- BRCA carrier, 1st degree relative with BRCA, 20% lifetime risk based on models, history of chest XRT
- Malignant calcifications- casting (linear and branching) or pleomorphic (granular). Benign calcifications- popcorn-like (fibroadenoma), large rod-like (secretory), round eggshell (oil cysts), and dystrophic or coarse (fat necrosis)
- BRCA
    - Tumor suppressor gene
    - BRCA 2- breast, pancreatic, and prostate cancer. Male has 6% breast cancer risk
    - BRCA 1 & 2 lifetime breast cancer risk is 50-85%
- ↑ progesterone receptors in the breast tissue- ↑ risk of breast cancer
- 2% risk of cancer in DCIS patient with skin-sparing mastectomy
- Boundaries of mastectomy- clavicle, sternum, IMF, anterior border of lat dorsi

- Breast cancer patient with large breasts- if partial mastectomy is required do reduction mammoplasty
- No nipple-sparing mastectomy if tumor >3 cm, <2 cm of the nipple, multicentric disease, + retroareolar frozen section, nodal disease
- Periareolar incisions for NSM only 25-50% of circumference
- ADM allows a greater initial fill of saline
- Medial pectoral nerve- inferior pectoralis + pec minor
- 2nd intercostobrachial nerve- skin of the axilla & inner arm
- Lateral intercostal nerve- breast
- 4th intercostal nerve- NAC
- Long thoracic- serratus anterior (winged scapula)
- Thoracodorsal- lat dorsi
- Latissimus dorsi flap
    - ↓ shoulder extension, adduction; hypertrophy of teres major
    - Place autologous skin paddle inferior, lateral
    - 35-60% seroma rate
    - Extended lat dorsi flap- includes scapular fascia & lumbar fat for additional volume. Can be used without implant
- Ryan flap- advancing lower thoracic tissue for breast reconstruction. Defines IMF. Good color match, easy, only IMF scar
- SIEA flap- lowest level of abdominal morbidity
- SGAP flap- firm consistency of gluteal fat. Difficult to mold for breasts
- Transverse musculocutaneous gracilis (TMG)- reconstruct small/medium breast
- ↓ flap loss with pedicled TRAM vs. free TRAM flap
- Bipedicled TRAM- vascular circulation to umbilicus is small vessels of the ligamentum teres
- If TRAM and lat dorsi fail, perform gluteus free flap
- Contralateral TRAM flap if defect of sternum, IMA, ribs, entire breast
- Venous congestion after DIEP with patent anastomosis- anastomose superficial venous system SIEV = supercharge flap
- Omental flap with skin graft- unnecessary abdominal procedure, no shaping of breast mound. Good in contaminated defect
- SGAP flap- a free sensate flap with abundance of adipose tissue, long pedicle, discrete scar, good projection, preserves gluteus muscle, low donor site morbidity
- Transverse upper gracilis (TUG) flap- upper inner thigh skin & subcutaneous tissues. Based on gracilis vessels & medial femoral circumflex artery, off from profunda femoris
- Breast reconstruction smokers- ↑ rate of mastectomy skin loss, donor site & umbilical necrosis, hernias
- Breast reconstruction & XRT
    - Autologous tissue is best
    - Tissue expander reconstruction can be done for XRT patients who refuse autologous reconstruction, but with ↑complications
    - Radiated tissue has vessel thrombosis
    - Redness & telangiectasias are not infection. Do not give antibiotics

- - o Late radiation effect- tissue deterioration, ↓vascularity, fibrosis, ulceration. Biopsy to rule out cancer
    - o Better to XRT then flap, otherwise flap will distort, shrink, fibrose
  - Treat minor infection without exposure of the prosthesis with antibiotics
  - Self-filling osmotic tissue expanders- no external fillings, ↓ risk of infection, no painful injections, filling phase of 40-60 days, require submuscular placement of a permanent prosthesis at 6 months
  - Venous outflow obstruction- ↑capillary refill, bluish skin, edema. Doppler may be normal. Rx- OR
  - Fat grafting corrects contour deformities in breast reconstruction
  - Liposuction improves lymphedema after axillary dissection

11. Breast Reduction

- Breast hypertrophy- due to abnormal end-organ responsiveness to estrogen. Normal estrogen levels and # receptors
- Skin flaps- 2 cm thick, preserve dermis
- Inferior pedicle Wise pattern- large, ptotic breasts
- Liposuction for breast reduction- minimal scars, rapid return to activity, ↓ operative time, normal sensation, ability to breast-feed. Disadvantages- not effective in young patients with dense breasts, difficult to assess amount of breast tissue removed, no path exam, poor skin shrinkage. Ideal patient- good skin elasticity, minimal hypertrophy, no ptosis
- Lateral, inferior & medial-based pedicles- better preservation of the nerve supply. Superior techniques- ↑nerve injury
- New nipple position determined with patient in an upright position pre-op. IMF most important landmark for nipple position
- Post-op NAC loss- pedicle torsion or tension. >5% occurrence. Early-reexplore pedicle. Consider making into free composite graft by grafting to well-vascularized, deepithelialized dermis. Late- wound care & delayed nipple reconstruction
- Free nipple grafting- ↓ necrosis in pts with >1500g resection, nipple transposition length >25cm, smoking, diabetes. Breast feeding not possible
- Superior quadrant skin is most sensitive & nipple is least sensitive to light pressure. Vibration is most sensitive in areola
- Post-op complication RF- ↑ BMI, volume >1000g per breast, tobacco
- Intraoperative hypotension results in higher rate of post-op hematoma
- Wound healing complications- young, healthy, obese patient with ↑ resection volumes
- Fat necrosis- hard, nontender lump 6 weeks post-op
- Scarring is MC source of patient dissatisfaction. Bottoming out, excessive or inadequate reduction, loss of sensation also complaints
- 27-35% of post-reduction patients breast feed
- Resection weight doesn't correlate with symptom relief

14

- ↑ complications with ↑ resection weight
- Mammogram findings post-op: parenchymal redistribution, elevation of the nipple, calcifications, retroareolar fibrotic banding, oil cysts
- Occult breast carcinoma in 2% reduction mammoplasty patients
- If tumor not completely excised during reduction mammaplasty, Rx-mastectomy

12. Facelift

- Improves static facial rhytids & nasolabial folds
- Aging skin histology- flat or separated dermal-epidermal junction; ↓ Langerhans cells, Type III collagen, ground substance; disorganization of extracellular matrix
- SMAS layers- galea, superficial temporal fascia, SMAS, platysma, superficial cervical fascia (facial nerve underneath). Continuous with parotid masseteric fascia
- Marionette lines caused by volume deflation & intact mandibular ligaments
- Midface access- temporal, blepharoplasty, or preauricular incision
- Midface lift corrects descended lid-cheek junction when done with lateral canthopexy of lower eyelid
- MACS lift- short scar facelift. Vertical vector only. SMAS purse-string sutured to deep temporal fascia
- Malar ptosis correction- elevate malar fat & suture to the deep temporal fascia
- If > 2cm fat pad advancement- disrupt angular vessels & necrosis can develop
- Malar implant- masseter muscle posterior, malar eminence superior, nasal labial fold medial
- Bevel the temporal incision to cut hair root at variable levels. May lead to better scar
- Secondary facelift patient- MC comorbidity is depression. Less skin excised. More likely to distort hair line, so use new incision
- MC facelift complication- hematoma. Rx- evacuation. Prevent- control BP, avoid aspirin, ginkgo, garlic, vitamin E
- Early motor nerve dysfunction- local anesthetic. Late- traction, cautery, sutures, transection
- MC facial nerve branch injured in facelift- buccal. Not noticeable, early return of function. Possibly unable to elevate one side of upper lip (levator labii oris muscle)
- Cervical branch injury- lower lip depressor weakness (like marginal mandibular branch) but mentalis & orbicularis normal
- Marginal mandibular nerve- variable location. 1-2cm below mandible. Injury- weakness of ipsilateral lip depressors (makes contralateral lower lip appears lower when smiling); weakness of mentalis & orbicularis oris (asymmetry with pursing of lips). Long term MM nerve paralysis Rx- local anesthetic block of contralateral depressor labii inferioris muscle (if this results in symmetry, use botox long-term)

Flap/wound interview delay (handwritten margin note)

I innervated superficial surface mentalis, Buccinator. Levator labii superioris (handwritten note)

15

- Frontal branch of facial nerve- motor, no sensory
- Great auricular nerve- travels superficial to platysma with EJ over SCM to lower posterior ear. Supplies helix, antihelix, cranial surface of ear
- Auriculotemporal nerve- branch of T3. Enters ear near tragus. Supplies tragus & helical root
- Greater occipital nerve- branch of C2-3. Supplies posterior scalp
- Lesser occipital nerve- branch of C2. Supplies upper 1/3 ear
- Spinal accessory nerve injury- shoulder pain, trapezius palsy, drooping shoulder, scapular winging. MC- iatrogentic. Located in posterior triangle of neck. Dx- EMG, nerve conduction studies. Rx- physical therapy & monitor 3 months, then if no improvement explore, neurolysis, repair, or grafting
- Vagus nerve- Arnold branch supplies concha
- Supraorbital nerve- superficial branch- central forehead sensation, deep branch-frontoparietal scalp sensation
- Supratrochlear nerve- nasal radix sensation. At risk during corrugator muscle resection
- Auriculotemporal & zygomaticotemporal nerve- temporal scalp sensation
- Transverse rhytids on root of nose Rx- procerus muscle resection. Origin- upper lateral cartilage & nasal bones, insertion- skin & glabella
- Buccal fat pad pseudoherniation- weak buccopharyngeal membrane. Small, reducible lower cheek mass. Rx- intraoral excision
- Neck rejuvenation evaluation- assess skin laxity, pre- & subplatysmal fat, position of chin, hyoid bone, thyroid cartilage. Ideal cervicomental angle is 105-120°
- Excess preplatysmal fat causes >120° cervicomental angle
- Neck bands- platysma separation. Rx- Plication laterally & midline
- Tissue sealants ↓ ecchymosis, edema, seroma, induration
- No evidence that steroids ↓facial swelling

13. Browlift
- Forehead- 1/3 facial length, 6-10 cm
- Ideal eyebrow- lower position medially, peaks from lateral-central limbus, descends at lateral orbital wall
- Endoscopic browlift- avoid recurrence of glabellar lines by removing all the muscle fibers of glabella between frontal bone & subcutaneous plane. Retains scalp sensation, normal forehead length.
- Pretrichial browlift incision shortens forehead, use for deep rhytides
- Coronal browlift incision- lengthens forehead, use on short forehead
- Transpalpebral corrugator resection- use when no eyebrow ptosis

14. Hair Transplant

- Hair production- matrix cell proliferation at base of hair follicle, then displaced, matures, produces keratin
- Transplanted hair unit- hair follicles with dermal elements. Good donor site- occipital scalp hair has longest lifespan   Donor Dominance
- Hair follicles located within subcutaneous layer of scalp
- Micrografting- hair growth for 1 month, then hair loss, then normal growth at 3 months
- Micro & minigrafts- healthy tissue has 95% take, scarred tissue has 85% take
- Balding- ↓ anagen phase, ↑ telogen phase. Anagen (active) phase- 3 years in men, 2-5 years longer in women. 90% of hair is in anagen phase
- Male-pattern hair loss- X-linked dominant gene. 60-80% of whites. Rx- scalp reduction. Sagittal excision removes greatest amount of bald skin, then re-establish anterior hairline
- Female-pattern hair loss- androgenetic alopecia. Loss at crown, preservation of frontal hairline. Some patients are hyperandrogenic- irregular menses, acne, hirsutism, PCOS
- Chronic telogen effluvium (telogen hair shedding)- causes female hair loss. Due to childbirth, malnutrition, infection, surgery, or mental stress. Growing hair shifts into resting (telogen) phase, then weeks to months later shedding begins. Self-limited. Hair restoration is unsuccessful & may worsen alopecia
- Psoriasis & tinea capitis- scaling, crusting scalp.
- Trichotillomania- traction alopecia from compulsive hair pulling
- Alopecia totalis- total hair loss over the entire scalp
- Alopecia areata- recurrent hair loss. Autoimmune. Rx- intralesional steroids, minoxidil. Hair loss is temporary or permanent
- Traction alopecia- trauma from hairstyle. Will grow back
- Anagen effluvium- insult to hair follicle that impairs metabolic activity. Example-chemotherapy. Results in tapered fracture of hair shafts
- Finasteride (propecia)- 5-alpha reductase enzyme to treat male pattern baldness
- IPL hair removal- destroys hair follicles using thermal injury to melanin-containing cells of the bulb
- Eyebrow missing from trauma- composite graft from scalp. Hair transplant unreliable

15. Rhinoplasty

- Nose functions- respiration, humidification, temperature regulation, particulate filtration, olfaction & phonation.
- 1/3 lobular portion, 2/3 columellar portion on worm's eye view. Nostrils- teardrop with long axis of nostril pointing medial
- Angle of divergence- middle crura of lower lateral cartilages
- Middle meatus- primary pathway of inspiratory nasal current

17

- Internal nasal valve borders- septum, upper lateral cartilage, pyriform aperture & inferior turbinate. Narrowest portion- 50% of nasal airway resistance
- Narrow internal nasal valve (<10°)- airway obstruction. Rx- butterfly grafts, flaring sutures, splay grafts & spreader grafts
- External nasal valve borders- caudal edge lower lateral cartilage, ala, septum & nostril sill
- External nasal valve collapse- weakening of lower lateral cartilage. Rx- alar batten grafts strengthen lateral crus of lower lateral cartilage
- Facial paralysis- nasal airway dysfunction due to collapse of external valve (levator labii superioris muscle)
- Lateral nasal artery- branch off anterior ethmoid, ICA. Blood supply to tip after division of columella
- Columellar artery- branch of superior labial, ECA. Blood supply to columella
- Angular artery- limit dissection above alar groove
- Sphenopalatine artery- posterior nasal septum
- Superior labial artery- upper lip
- Posterior ethmoid artery- upper central nasal septum
- Anterior ethmoid nerve- nasal tip & lateral nasal vault
- Infraorbital nerve- lateral nose, ala, columella
- Infratrochlear nerve- upper nasal sidewalls & skin over radix
- Supraorbital nerve- skin over radix
- Supratrochlear nerve- forehead
- Nasopalatine nerve- inferior septum. Travels from pterygopalatine ganglion, through incisive foramen, joins greater palatine nerve
- Internal nasal nerve- branch of anterior ethmoid nerve. Supplies anterior nasal lining
- Lesser palatine nerve- soft palate sensation
- Traumatic deviation of nasal septum- examine septum, ethmoid & vomer
- Septoplasty- preserve 1-cm L strut to preserve internal nasal valve
- L-strut fracture- will rotate posteriorly, resulting in a saddle-nose deformity. Rx- spreader grafts to secure the L-strut in place
- Septal perforation- bleeding, whistling. Rx- flap, graft
- Saddle-nose deformity- collapsed dorsum. May be due to septal hematoma, excessive resection of nasal dorsum or septum, fracture of perpendicular plate of ethmoid or nasal bones during infracture. Rx- onlay cartilage or bone graft
- Inverted-V deformity- excessive removal of transverse portion of upper lateral cartilage. Rx- spreader grafts
- Boxy tip deformity- due to lower lateral cartilage position. Angle of divergence of middle crura determines intercrural distance. Ideal- 30-60°. Wide angle (>90°) domes appear like corners of a box
- Open roof deformity- taking down dorsal hump. Rx- infracture or spreader graft
- Pollybeak deformity- scar causing tip fullness that pushes it down
- Rocker deformity- medial osteotomy of nasal bones goes beyond radix, distal portion rocks lateral

- Alar notching- over-resection of lower lateral cartilages
- Supratip deformity Rx- steroid injection within 3 months post-op if due to scar between dorsum & skin
- Middle nasal vault collapse- prevent by using spreader grafts
- Spreader grafts- Rx internal nasal valve, deviated septum, open roof deformity
- Weir excisions- resection of the alar bases to reduce wide, flaring nostrils
- Hanging columella Rx- resection of the caudal septum
- Wide nasal bridge Rx- osteotomy of frontal process of maxilla
- Dorsal hump Rx- dorsal implant, hump rasping or resection, osteotomy & nasal bone infracture
- Infracture of the nasal bones- narrows nasal dorsum. Narrowing internal nasal valve can cause breathing difficulties
- Full-transfixion incision- ↓ tip projection if dissected over anterior nasal spine because loss of nasal tip support. Rx- columellar strut
- External perforating osteotomy- at nasofacial junction, avoid angular artery
- Transdomal suture- narrows the domes & lateral crura, ↑ tip projection. Use for broad, bulbous tip
- Interdomal suture- use if asymmetrical domal height, or to ↓ interdomal width
- Columellar septal suture- establish tip strength
- Lateral crural mattress suture- makes lateral crural concavity
- Medial crural sutures- ↓ or ↑ tip projection
- ↑ nasal tip projection- cartilage graft, medial crura sutures or strut graft
- Pinched nasal tip Rx- alar grafts
- Crural turnover graft- supports weakened or deformed lower lateral cartilages
- Spring graft- spans the upper lateral cartilages. Widens the middle vault
- Thick skin & prominent sebaceous glands- harder to achieve smaller nasal tip
- Open rhinoplasty technique- may place columellar strut if unstable
- Post-op anosmia test- trigeminal nervous system still recognizes ammonia. Used to diagnose malingering
- Cottle maneuver- lateral traction on cheek skin displaces lateral nasal wall, opening internal nasal valve
- Rhinomanometry- evaluate nasal cavity patency & air passage
- Nasal bone fractures- 3 zones
  - Upper vault- nasal bones, ethmoid, vomer, cephalic septal border
  - Middle vault- upper lateral cartilages, septum, maxilla
  - Lower vault- alar cartilages, inferior septum. Rx- upper & middle vault- septum & nasal bones reduction, spreader grafts
- Post-op white spot on tip of nose- pressure on nasal tip from graft

- Soft-tissue fillers to use in nose- hyaluronic acid-derived & calcium hydroxyapatite. Do no use silicone. Place just above periosteum to ↓ visibility & palpability. Use only on dorsum & sidewalls
- Periostitis of the nasal dorsum- post-op nasal dorsum redness due to retained rasping shavings. Rx- antibiotics, resect dorsal prominence in 1 year. Prevent- irrigation
- Asian nose- alar flare, bulbous tip, short columella, thick subcutaneous tissue & wide, flat nasal dorsum, shorter height of upper & lower lateral cartilages
- Congenital choanal atresia- bone or soft tissue blockage presenting shortly after birth
- Nasal tip droops with old age due to loss of lower lateral cartilage support
- Surgical antibiotic prophylaxis- ancef 1g for most plastic surgery procedures. If allergy, give clindamycin
- Perioperative steroid use ↓ edema & ecchymosis of upper & lower eyelids after blepharoplasty & nose after rhinoplasty. Multiple, tapered dosing starting pre-op is best
- Body dysmorphic disorder- 7-15% of plastic surgery patients. MC-nose. Preoccupied >1hr per day & impairs social function. No relationship to sex or marital status
- SIMON- single, immature male, overly narcissistic
- Numb nasal tip post-op- injury to external branch of anterior ethmoidal nerve. MC- endonasal rhinoplasty procedures

16. Chin

- Witch's chin deformity- complication of genioplasty lower buccal sulcus incision with mentalis muscle division. Prevent- leave cuff of muscle to help close
- Post-genioplasty lip paresthesia- resolves in 2-3 weeks. If not, remove & trim prosthesis in the area of mental nerve foramen
- Augmentation genioplasty implant to skin ratio is around 0.8. (example: 6mm deficiency treated with 7mm implant)
- Porous polyethylene facial prostheses are less likely to migrate than silicone due to tissue ingrowth
- Silicone prosthesis adds sagittal projection to pogonion
- Osseous genioplasty treats vertical deficiency
- Medpor prosthesis will vertically lengthen chin, smooth labial mental fold, add sagittal projection

17. Cosmetic Chemicals, Fillers & Peels

- Fitzpatrick skin types
  - I (white)- always burns
  - II (white)- usually burns

- o III (white)- average tan
- o IV (white)- rarely burns
- o V (brown)- tans easily
- o VI (black)- never burns
- Botox
  - o MOA- inhibition of the release of acetylcholine
  - o paralysis 3-7 days until 4-6 months
  - o only FDA-approved for glabellar area → *glabella c̄ crows feet*
  - o Treat glabellar wrinkles with 20U
  - o Eyelid drooping- inhibition of frontalis muscle or diffusion through orbital septum to levator muscle. Rx- α-adrenergic eye drops (iopidine), which contracts Mueller's muscle
  - o Rx for platysmal banding to avoid neck lift or platysmaplasty. Don't inject below thyroid cartilage
  - o ↑ effect: penicillamine, quinine, calcium-channel blockers & aminoglycosides
  - o Anticholinesterase (pyridostigmine) counteracts effects until Botox wears off
  - o Indications- cervical dystonia, axillary hyperhidrosis, strabismus, blepharospasm
- Dysport- botulinum toxin to reduce glabellar furrows. Contraindicated for patients with cow's milk allergy
- Myobloc- botox-resistant patients. More pain with injection
- Eyebrow elevation- frontalis. Depression- orbicularis oculi, corrugator supercilii, depressor supercilii & procerus. Bunny lines- nasalis. Glabellar lines- corrigator. Crow's feet- orbicularis oculi. Horizontal nasal lines- procerus.
- Fillers
  - o Hyaluronic acid injectables (Juvéderm, Restylane, Perlane)- ↑ fullness in nasolabial fold & lip area
  - o Restylane- highest concentration of hyaluronic acid
  - o Inject at the level of the periosteum when injecting hyaluronic acids for tear trough correction
  - o S/S of vascular compromise- pain, edema, bluish discoloration. Rx- massage, warm compresses, nitro paste, injection of hyaluronidase, HBO. Necrosis Rx- antibiotic ointment, debridement
  - o Zyplast, Zyderm- 3% of patients have allergic reaction due to bovine collagen allergy *— test dose*
- Rhytides Rx- first-line is retinoid, hydroquinone, or glycolic acids. Next is TCA peel
- Tretinoin- ↓ pigmentation & wrinkles due to ↓ melanin & ↑ transit rate of keratinocytes through the epidermis. Thins the stratum corneum, reverses cellular atypia, thickens the epidermis, ↑ collagen synthesis, hyaluronic acid & dermal mucin. Defer dermabrasion & laser resurfacing for 1 year. SE- erythema, photosensitivity & desquamation. Must wear sunscreen
- Isotretinoin- Accutane- impairs sebaceous gland activity & epithelialization, thins stratum corneum

↳ 1yr for any laser or dermabrasion or peel

21

- Dermabrasion- dermal-epidermal junction- smooth, doesn't bleed. Papillary dermis- sparse, punctate bleeding. Superficial reticular dermis- brisk bleeding, endpoint of treatment. Used for perioral rhytides, acne scarring, traumatic tattoos. Re-epithelization from hair follicles, sebaceous glands & sweat ducts. Less hypopigmentation, so use in patients with darker complexions. Do no use around the eye
- Jessner solution- resorcinol, salicylic acid & lactic acid. 14% each in ethanol. Destroys connections between keratinocytes, removes the epidermis, ↑ epidermal turnover, ↓ melanin
- Kojic acid- skin lightener that inhibits tyrosinase. Rx- melasma. SE- skin irritation, sun sensitivity
- Phenol peel- Rx- coarse wrinkles, severe sun damage & significant pigment problems. Depth decreased with liquid soap. SE- rare cardiac, severe hypopigmentation
- TCA peel- Rx- moderate facial rhytides. Neutralized in superficial dermal plexus by keratin
- 30% glycolic peel- short recovery period, penetrates to stratum corneum, results in mild epidermal peeling
- Hydroquinones- bleaching agent. Tyrosine kinase inhibitor blocks dopamine→ melanin
- Alpha-hydroxy acids- desquamation due to ↓ corneocyte cohesion, resulting in ↑ collagen & glycosaminoglycans
- Vitamin C- antioxidant that protects skin from UV radiation, ↑ collagen, ↓ pigment synthesis, improved epidermis
- Antiviral prophylaxis with acyclovir or valacyclovir in all peel patients to prevent herpes
- HIV lipoatrophy- only poly-L-lactic acid (Sculptra) is FDA-approved
- Fat grafting- 70% resorption over time. Place small amounts of fat with each pass at 90 degree lines. Prepare using balanced centrifugation
- Ice-pick scarring is full-thickness. Rx- direct excision
- Zinc oxide- effective against UVA & UVB. SPF is UVB only

18. Lasers

- KTP 532-595nm- superficial red vessels
- Pulsed-dye laser 585nm wavelength chromophore- oxyhemoglobin. Treats vascular lesions
- Q-switched Nd:YAG 1064nm- deepest penetration. Least risk of hypopigmentation but also least effective with brightly colored tattoos
- Nd:YAG 532nm- red, orange, yellow ink. SE- purpura x 1 wk
- Nd:YAG 1064nm- hair reduction, collagen stimulation, blue vessels
- Nd:YAG, diode, erbium lasers- wavelengths 1064-1540nm. Best for acne scars
- Q-switched lasers (ruby, Nd:YAG, alexandrite) are based on select photothermolysis Removes black & color tattoo pigments, homemade tattoos. Minimal scar. SE- transient hypopigmentation
- Pulsed-dye laser with epidermal cooling- port-wine stains

- Fractionated carbon dioxide laser chromophore- water. Treats rhytides, acne scars, dyschromias
- Acne can occur post-laser treatment
- Erythema can last up to 4 months post-laser treatment. CO_2 > fractionated CO_2 or Er:YAG. Rx- topical ascorbic acid ↓ duration & severity
- Post-laser scarring Rx- topical or intralesional steroids, silicone sheets, pulsed-dye laser
- Pigmented skin (Fitzpatrick III or IV) absorbs more laser energy than nonpigmented skin. Thermal damage extends beyond treatment area. MC SE- hyperpigmentation, Rx- hydroquinone, tretinoin, avoid sun. Pretreat with retinoic acid or bleaching agents to avoid hyperpigmentation. Usually resolves within a few months
- Isotretinoin (Accutane) contraindicated for any skin resurfacing procedure
- Antiviral prophylaxis used in all patients undergoing laser resurfacing
- Viral, bacterial & fungal infections can develop after laser resurfacing. MC- HSV2. Rx- acyclovir 2 days before until 10 days after
- Systemic herpetic infection S/S- cutaneous lesions, shortness of breath, fever, chills, malaise, headache, neurologic changes. Rx- IV antivirals & antibiotics

19. Craniofacial

- Suture closing- metopic suture- 6 months, sagittal suture- 22 years, coronal suture- 24 years, lambdoid suture- 26 years, squamosal suture- 35 years
- Posterior fontanelle closes by 2 months. Anterior fontanelle closes by 18-24 months
- Metopic synostosis- trigonocephaly, midline forehead prominence, orbital narrowing, bilateral parietal widening, hypotelorism, abnormalities of corpus callosum & developmental delays. Isolated metopic ridge can be normal. Head shape determines surgical need
- Coronal synostosis- unilateral flattening of forehead, deviation of nasal root, flattening of occiput, widening of palpebral fissure, superior & posterior displacement of supraorbital rim & eyebrow, higher ear. Anterior fontanelle is displaced away from affected side. Low orbital roof causes strabismus- child tilts head, covering the affected eye resolves. FGFR3 mutation on chromosome 4p16. Rx- fronto-orbital advancement
- Harlequin deformity- X-ray opacity from inferior/medial to superior/lateral through orbital aperture. Due to superior displacement of lesser wing of sphenoid from coronal synostosis
- Sagittal synostosis- scaphocephaly. Elongated head. Rx- endoscopic correction- synostectomy of fused suture, microfracturing of parietal bones & postoperative orthotic at 2-4 months old
- Lambdoid synostosis- occipitoparietal flattening, ipsilateral mastoid bulge. Posterior ear. Rx- posterior vault expansion, remodeling

23

- Deformational plagiocephaly- parallelogram-shaped skull, anterior ear
- Kleeblattschädel skull deformity- multiple suture synostoses. ↑ ICP. Moth-eaten. Rx- early surgery
- Orbital hypertelorism- ↑ interorbital distance measured from dacryon (the junction of the frontal, lacrimal & maxillary bones) to dacryon. Normal is 28mm-men, 25mm- women
- Pseudohypertelorism- aka telecanthus. ↑ intercanthal distance, but normal interorbital distance.
- Hypotelorism- ↓ intraorbital distance. From trigonocephaly of metopic synostosis
- Exotropia- eyes deviate outward
- Esotropia- eyes deviate inward
- Exophthalmos- globe protrusion due to ↑ orbital contents in normal bony orbit
- Enophthalmos- globe recessed in orbit due to ↑ bony volume. Traumatic or surgical malposition
- Exorbitism- globe protrusion due to ↓ capacity of bony orbit (seen in hypertelorism, Apert)
- Vertical maxillary excess- long-face deformity- long lower 1/3 of face. Lip incompetence, long retruded chin, gummy smile, flat mid-face, obtuse nasolabial angle, narrow alar bases, class II malocclusion, anterior open bite. Rx- Le Fort I osteotomy, superior repositioning of maxilla, genioplasty
- Normal maxillary incisor show- 2-3 mm
- Verticle maxillary deficiency- short lower 1/3 of face, class II malocclusion, ↑ SNA, SNB angles. Rx- Lefort I with downward positioning
- Maxillary retrusion- hypoplasia, ↓ vertical height, class III malocclusion. ↓ SNA, ↑ SNB angle. Rx- Lefort II
- Mandibular retrusion- retrusive chin, class II malocclusion
- Mandibular excess- no retrusive chin, class III malocclusion
- McCune-Albright syndrome- fibrous dysplasia, precocious puberty, cafe-au-lait spots. Rx- pamidronate ↓ bone pain
- Klippel-Feil syndrome- fusion of cervical vertebrae, short neck, low occipital hairline & restricted spine mobility
- Paget disease of the bone- osteitis deforman. Large, deformed bones. Dx- alk phos
- Treacher Collins syndrome- AD. Hypoplasia of zygoma, maxilla, mandible, ear abnormalities, lower eyelid coloboma, preauricular hair displacement, downward slant of palpebral fissures, no eyelashes. Gene TCOF1. Complete form- no malar bone or zygomatic arch
- Pierre Robin sequence- micrognathia or retrognathia, glossoptosis, airway obstruction (+/- CP). Rx- prone position, upright feedings, NG tube, intubation, tongue-lip adhesion. Surgery- mandibular distraction with nasoendoscopy pre-op to rule out laryngomalacia, webbing
- Stickler syndrome- ocular problems (retinal detachment, myopia, blindness), facial abnormalities (flat nose, small mandible, CP), hearing loss, degenerative joint disease, pain. 40% of Pierre Robin patients

poly ostotic s
fibrous dysplasia

40% have Pierre Robin

24

- Apert syndrome- AD. Bicoronal craniosynostosis (turribrachycephaly), midface hypoplasia, hand & feet syndactyly *exorb. h?*
- Crouzon syndrome- AD. Craniosynostosis of coronal, sagittal & lambdoid sutures (turribrachycephaly), midface hypoplasia, exorbitism, proptosis, normal extremities *upper Aperts*
- Crouzon, Apert, and Pfeiffer syndromes- bicoronal synostosis, hypoplastic mid face *↳ lower Aperts*
- Goldenhar syndrome- oculoauriculovertebral dysplasia. Asymmetry of hard & soft facial tissues that is usually unilateral. Mandibular hypoplasia, epibulbar dermoids, microtia, vertebral & ear abnormalities. Epibulbar dermoids distinguishes from hemifacial microsomia
- Nager syndrome- acrofacial dysostosis. AR. Hypoplasia of orbits, zygoma, maxilla, mandible, soft palate, auricular defects, hypoplasia of radius, thumbs, metacarpals, radioulnar synostosis, elbow joint deformities *Ear defect ⊕ upper extremity*
- Sturge-Weber syndrome- port-wine stain in V1 or V2 distribution
- Van der Woude syndrome- AD. Lower lip pits, CL/CP, hypodontia, high arched palate. IRF6 gene
- Mobius syndrome- congenital facial weakness, abnormal ocular abduction, weakness of CN VI & VII, mask-like facial appearance, abducens nerve paralysis. Rx- strabismus surgery to correct paralysis of lateral gaze. 25% have limb abnormalities. Other CN may be involved
- Romberg disease- aka progressive hemifacial atrophy. Hypoplasia of maxilla & mandible, dental disturbances, seizures, migraines, Horner syndrome, hemiplegia. Coup de sabre- classic early sign in 50% of patients. Unknown cause. 1st-2nd decade. Trigeminal dermatome. Rx- immunosuppression(?). Rx- implants, fillers, bone grafts, fat grafts, free tissue transfer (parascapular flap)
- Velocardiofacial syndrome- deletion on chromosome 22. Disruption of neural crest cell development. CP, VPI, cardiac abnormalities. Broad nose, malar flattening, epicanthal folds, retrognathia, vertical maxillary excess, absence of the thymus and parathyroid glands. MRA may show medicalization of carotid artery before palatal or pharyngeal surgery. Dx- FISH analysis
- Saethre-Chotzen syndrome- acrocephalosyndactyly. Coronal craniosynostosis, low hairline, proptosis, antimongoloid slanting of palpebral fissures, nasal deviation. No CP
- Albright syndrome- AD. Calcium & phosphate metabolism issues. Low nasal bridge, short neck
- Binder syndrome- midface retrusion, nasomaxillary hypoplasia, convex lip, short nose, flat frontonasal angle, no anterior nasal spine, hypoplastic frontal sinuses. Due to anterior nasal floor hypoplasia. Rx- surgery to ↑ nose length & projection- Le Fort I & II osteotomy, orthodontics, bone & cartilage grafts
- Carpenter syndrome- AR. Brachycephaly from variable synostoses, cardiovascular, musculoskeletal & genital defects
- Down syndrome- trisomy 21. Craniofacial manifestations- brachycephaly, low nasal bridge, epicanthal folds

- 22q deletion syndrome- DiGeorge, velocardiofacial & Shprintzen syndromes. Congenital heart disease, CP, learning disabilities, long facial features, teenage mental illness, calcium regulation issues
- CHARGE syndrome- coloboma, heart defects, nasal choanae atresia, growth retardation, genital abnormalities, ear abnormalities
- Ectodermal dysplasia- X-linked recessive. Hypoplastic skin & ↓ dermal appendages
- Neurofibromatosis 1- neurofibromas, optic gliomas. Plexiform neurofibromas- grow along nerves, involves multiple fascicles & branches. ~10% risk of malignant peripheral nerve sheath tumor arising from pre-existing neurofibroma
- Craniofacial microsomia- 2nd MC head/neck congenital anomaly after CL/CP. Caused by intrauterine event, not genetic. Multiple anomalies- mandible> ear> vertebrae> ribs> ipsilateral facial nerve> genitourinary. VPI common in hemifacial microsomia due to unilateral hypodynamic palate. Macrostomia, 1st branchial cleft sinus, cranial nerve abnormalities. Multiple surgeries- macrostomia repair in few months after birth, skeletal & soft-tissue repair at 5 years
- Tessier Clefts
    - 3- orbit. Unilateral CL, ala, medial canthus, colobomas medial to punctum, lacrimal gland anomalies. Bone- alveolus between lateral incisor & canine
    - 4- lateral to cupid's bow to the nasolacrimal canal. Bone- between lateral incisor & canine, medial to infraorbital foramen
    - 5- CL, lower eyelid coloboma. Bone- canine, maxillary sinus to orbital floor
    - 6- incomplete Treacher Collins syndrome. Oral commissure toward the angle of mandible, lower eyelid coloboma
    - 7- macrostomia. Incomplete merging of mandibular & maxillary prominences of 1st pharyngeal arch. Varies in severity involving oral commissure, sideburns, external ear. Bone- zygomatic arch, maxillary second molar. Can also have duplicated maxilla, supranumery teeth
    - 8- inferior displacement of lateral canthi
- MC cleft is #7, least common is #9
- Failed merging with maxillary prominence- Tessier 2, 3 or 4 facial cleft
- TMJ- assess motion by placing fingers inside or anterior to ear canal. Clicking- subluxation of articular disk between the two joint spaces. Rx- splint, NSAIDS, PT
- Dermoid cysts- slow-growing mass on lateral brow or midline glabellar region. Assess intracranial communication with CT or MRI
- Encephalocele- soft, mobile midline malformation present at birth that changes size with crying. Broadens nasal root, ↑ intercanthal distance. US- occipital, Asia- frontoethmoidal Prognosis- presence or absence of herniated brain tissue. Rx- early excision.
- Glioma- neural tissue left during embryonic development. Broadens nasal root, ↑ intercanthal distance

- Rathke pouch- ectoderm invaginates toward hypophysis. Cyst located in nasopharynx
- Distraction osteogenesis- fibrous zone- central area with fibrous tissue; transitional zone-fibrous tissue undergoing ossification, zone of remodeling bone, zone of mature bone.
- Le Fort III osteotomy- correct midface deficiency, malocclusion
- Distraction osteogenesis better than bone grafting for >10mm advancement- less relapse, gradual stretching of soft-tissue envelope, ↓ morbidity, less secondary procedures
- Midfacial advancement- ↓ SNB, ↑ ANB, ↓ negative overjet, ↑ upper airway volume (improves obstructive sleep apnea)

20. Cleft Lip & Palate

- Fusion of the medial nasal, lateral nasal & maxillary prominences produces the nose, upper lip & palate. MNP- nasal tip, columella, philtrum, premaxilla, downgrowth forms nasal septum. FNP- bridge of nose, forehead. LNP- nasal ala
- Primary CP- unsuccessful fusion of median & lateral palatine processes. Secondary CP-unsuccessful fusion of lateral palatine processes to each other & nasal septum
- CL- failure of fusion of maxillary prominence & MNP
- Embryonic period of anomalies- CL wks 5-6, CP wks 7-8, eye & ear wks 10-12
- Anatomy of cleft- bony septum deviated to cleft side, anterior nasal spine deviated to noncleft side, ↓ sagittal projection of the pyriform sinus, dentoalveolar arch
- Veau classification
  - Class I- incomplete cleft of soft palate
  - Class II- hard & soft palate, but limited to secondary palate
  - Class III- complete unilateral CL/P
  - Class IV- complete bilateral CL/P
- Inheritance patterns-
Family Members	CL & CL/P	CP
One child with deformity	4%	2%
One parent with deformity	4%	6%
One parent & one child with deformity	17%	15%
Two children with deformity	9%	
- Associated anomalies - CL/P 10%. CP 50%
- Lateral incisor is MC tooth affected by CL/P
- Submucous cleft palate- bifid uvula, hard palate notch, zona pellucida. Anomalous insertion of levator muscles onto posterior hard palate. Usually asymptomatic, but may have VPI, hypernasal speech
- CP repair- desire separation of oral & nasal cavities, repair levator musculature for normal speech (intravelar veloplasty)
- Treat VPI at age 4 for hypernasality

levator veli
palatini
CN X

tensor veli
palatini
CN V

- Pharyngeal flap- treats VPI. Elevate a rectangular flap, based superiorly or inferiorly, from posterior pharynx & inset into soft palate. Width based on lateral pharyngeal wall motion
- Sphincter pharyngoplasty- treats VPI from large-gap or poor lateral wall motion. Elevate tonsillar pillar (palatopharyngeus muscle) superior, rotate 90° medial, sew into posterior pharyngeal wall at the adenoid   CN X
- Palatal lift- enough tissue, but poor coordination
- Preoperative gap size is best predictor of outcome after VPI surgery
- Obturator- used when inadequate palatal tissue
- Repair levator veli palatini to improve eustachian tube function
- Nasoalveolar molding- intraoral appliance that narrows the cleft, aligns the segments, shapes the nose. Stents can be used for columella lengthening
- Complete unilateral CL- ala displaced laterally, inferiorly, posteriorly
- CL repair- A flap- medial lip rotation flap. B flap- non-cleft, lateral lip advancement flap. L flap- lateral lip used for nasal lining defect. M flap- medially based. C flap- lengthens columella
- Abbe flap- creates a philtrum in CL patients with upper lip tightness. Lower lip tissue replaces aesthetic subunit of upper lip. Pedicle (labial artery) divided at 2-4 wks
- Unrepaired alveolar cleft- posterior crossbite of maxillary dentition
- Class III malocclusion- maxillary retrusion & mandibular prognathism. Rx- maxillary advancement (Le Fort I) & sagittal split osteotomy (mandibular setback)
- Cephalometric x-ray used to determine completion of maxillofacial growth
- Tongue vasculature- paired lingual arteries run on lateral ventral 1/3 of tongue. Additional vascularity- facial, ascending pharyngeal arteries
- Tensor veli palatini muscle- from skull base to eustachian tube, around hamulus, then forms aponeurosis with contralateral muscle in soft palate
- Retrognathia- posterior displacement of chin with normal mandibular dimensions
- Microgenia- mental symphysis abnormally develops
- Palatopharyngeus muscle- CN XI through pharyngeal plexus
- Tensor veli palatini- medial pterygoid nerve
- Palate- greater & lesser palatine nerves
- Lingual muscles- hypoglossal nerve, except palatoglossus (vagus nerve)
- Van der Woude syndrome- AD. CL/P with lower lip pitting (accessory salivary glands)
- Pierre Robin sequence- glossoptosis, micrognathia or retrognathia, CP. Manage airway obstruction- place prone, intubate

tensor
veli
palatini
open
eustachian
tube

28

21. Head & Neck

- External carotid artery branches- superior thyroid, ascending pharyngeal, lingual, occipital, facial, posterior auricular, maxillary
- Stylomastoid foramen- facial nerve, foramen lacerum- ICA, foramen ovale- mandibular (V3) nerve, foramen rotundum- maxillary (V2) nerve, jugular foramen- glossopharyngeal, vagus & spinal accessory nerves Foramen rotundum- maxillary division of trigeminal nerve —> V2 (infraorbital nerve) V3
- Foramen ovale- mandibular division of trigeminal nerve, lesser petrosal branch of glossopharyngeal nerve, accessory meningeal branch of maxillary artery
- Foramen spinosum- meningeal branch of mandibular division of trigeminal nerve, middle meningeal artery & vein
- Tongue innervation- anterior 2/3 sensation- lingual nerve, mandibular division of trigeminal. Anterior 2/3 taste- chorda tympani of facial nerve. Posterior 1/3 tongue- glossopharyngeal. Motor nerve to tongue- hypoglossal
- Hypoglossal nerve- motor of ipsilateral intrinsic & most extrinsic muscle of tongue. Exception- palatoglossus (X)
- Supraorbital nerve- sensation of forehead, anterior & frontoparietal scalp. Preserve with bicoronal incision. Superficial branch travels superficial to frontalis muscle in forehead.
- Supratrochlear nerve- medial forehead sensation. Passes through corrugator muscle
- Sphenopalatine nerve- incisive foramen. Anterior hard palate sensation
- Lesser palatine nerve- greater palatine foramen. Soft palate & uvula sensation
- Glossopharyngeal nerve- parasympathetic to parotid gland, sensation of carotid body & sinus, posterior 1/3 tongue, external ear skin, tympanic membrane, taste for posterior 1/3 tongue
- Chorda tympani- parasympathetic to submandibular & sublingual
- Afferent chorda tympani- anterior 2/3 tongue taste
- Bell's palsy- block within meatal or labyrinthine segments, proximal to chorda tympani & stapedial nerves. Causes taste change & dampening of loud noises
- Trigeminal nerve- 1st- ophthalmic- sensory. 2nd- maxillary- sensory. 3rd- mandibular- mixed sensory & motor
- Maxillary nerve- sensation to ipsilateral face, nose, lip, upper teeth
- Vestibulocochlear nerve- CN VIII. Sound & equilibrium to brain
- Vagus nerve- palatoglossus, pharyngeal constrictors, uvulae, palatopharyngeus
- Arnold nerve- aka auricular branch of vagus, CN X. Innervates external acoustic meatus. Stimulation causes reflex coughing (Arnold reflex)
- Inferior alveolar nerve- enters medial ramus 10mm below sigmoid notch, exits anteriorly at 1st molar through mental foramen. Innervates lower lip & chin

CN VII

- Facial nerve- innervates face muscles on posterior surface. Exceptions- levator anguli oris, buccinator, mentalis. 1st branchial arch sinuses & cysts
- Frontal branch of facial nerve lies within superficial temporal (temporoparietal) fascia
- Buccal branch of facial nerve innervates buccinator, levator anguli oris, orbicularis oris, risorius
- Mandibular branch of facial nerve innervates depressor anguli oris
- External ear sensation- great auricular & lesser occipital nerves innervate posterior auricle & lobule. Auriculotemporal nerve innervates anterior ear- helix, scapha, concha (MC injured with trigeminal neuralgia decompression). Vagus & glossopharyngeal nerves innervate external auditory meatus
- Great auricular nerve- innervates 1st branchial arch structures. Auriculotemporal nerve- innervates 2nd branchial arch structures
- Auriculotemporal nerve block- blocks helix & tragus. Inject superior & anterior to tragus. Great auricular nerve & lesser occipital nerve block- blocks earlobe and lateral helix. Inject posterior sulcus at inferior earlobe
- Spinal accessory nerve- motor- SCM & trapezius
- Muscles of mastication- temporalis, masseter, medial & lateral pterygoids
- Buccinator muscle- only cheek compressor
- Buccinator & orbicularis oris- lip compressors
- Levator labii superioris, risorius, zygomaticus major- separate the lips. From bone & fascia to lips
- Masseter- from zygomatic arch to lateral ramus. Elevates the mandible
- Digastric muscle- mastoid process to hyoid bone & anterior mandible. Depresses mandible, elevates hyoid
- Masseter, medial pterygoid, temporalis- elevate mandible
- Medial pterygoid- from lateral pterygoid plate & tuberosity of maxilla to medial angle
- Depressor septi nasi muscle- cause nasal tip descent, upper lip shortening, transverse crease in philtrum. Origin- medial crura. Insert- incisive fossa of maxilla or orbicularis oris muscle. Rx- excision or botox
- Temporalis- from temporal fossa to coronoid process & anterior ramus
- Mylohyoid muscle- forms oral cavity floor. From mandible to hyoid bone. Elevates floor of mouth when swallowing, elevates hyoid bone & tongue, lowers mandible, opens mouth, mastication, sucking, blowing. Innervation- mylohyoid branch of inferior alveolar nerve of mandibular nerve
- Nasalis muscle- compresses nose, brings ala toward septum
- Risorius muscle- retracts angle of mouth (smile)
- Zygomaticus major muscle- brings angle of mouth posterior/superior (laughing)
- Tensor tympani muscle- attaches to malleus. Innervation- trigeminal nerve

- Tensor veli palatini muscle- from eustachian tube & medial pterygoid plate, around hamulus, into palate. Innervation- trigeminal nerve. Dilates eustachian tube
- Levator veli palatine- located in posterior palate. Elevates soft palate when swallowing or yawning. Innervation- vagus
- Palatoglossus muscles- form anterior tonsillar pillars, lift base of tongue, insert into uvula
- Digastric & stylohyoid muscles- cut for better exposure of carotid bifurcation
- 7 orbit bones- frontal, maxilla, zygoma, ethmoid, lacrimal, greater & lesser wings of sphenoid, palatine
- Lesser wing of sphenoid- posterior roof. Transmits optic nerve & ophthalmic artery in optic canal
- Greater wing of sphenoid- transmits lacrimal nerve, frontal nerve, trochlear nerve, superior & inferior branches of oculomotor nerve, nasociliary nerve, & abducens nerve in superior orbital fissure
- Maxillary sinus drains into middle meatus. Maxillary antrostomy- enlarging ostium & resecting uncinate process of ethmoid endoscopically
- Frontal sinus drains into middle meatus
- Posterior ethmoidal cells & sphenoidal sinus drain into superior meatus
- Layers- skin- subcutaneous tissue- superficial temporal fascia- superficial layer of deep temporal fascia- superficial temporal fat pad- deep layer of deep temporal fascia- temporalis muscle
- Coronal flap- include superficial layer of deep temporal fascia in the flap to protect frontal branch
- Superficial fascia- SCM, trapezius, suprahyoid muscles
- Prevertebral fascia- scalenes & paravertebral muscles
- Pretracheal fascia- thyroid & trachea
- Parotid papilla- Stensen's duct empties next to maxillary second molar
- Parotid duct- middle third of line between tragus & upper lip. Leaves anterior parotid gland, superficial to masseter, pierces buccinators, enters oral cavity opposite maxillary 2nd molar
- Thyroid gland- first endocrine gland to develop (starts at 24 days, done by 7 wks). From foramen cecum from 1st & 2nd pouches
- Berry ligament- attaches thyroid to laryngoskeleton. Causes thyroid gland to move during swallowing
- Thyroglossal duct cyst- failure of thyroglossal duct atrophy. Rx- resect central hyoid bone & cyst
- Lingual thyroid- failure of thyroid gland descent. Posterior tongue mass, airway obstruction
- Hyoid bone- ossification of 2nd & 3rd pharyngeal arch cartilage
- Ectopic thyroid gland- MC at base of tongue, posterior to foramen cecum
- Ectopic parathyroid gland- 15-20% of patients. Can be anywhere
- 1st arch- malleus, incus, maxilla, mandible, zygoma, mastication muscles, trigeminal nerve, external carotid artery

- 2nd arch- most arch abnormalities. Stapes, styloid, hyoid, face muscles, posterior digastric, facial nerve, palatine tonsils
- 2nd pharyngeal cleft & pouch anomalies- cyst, fistula, sinus. MC- cyst. Fistulas present at birth, opening @ anterior SCM, swallowing can cause puckering
- 3rd arch- stylopharyngeus, internal & common carotid arteries, ~~vagus~~ nerve

(margin note: VAGUS CN X)

- 4-6th arches- pharyngeal & laryngeal muscles, thyroid cartilage
- Branchial cleft sinus or fistula- embryologic remnant of the cleft between 2nd & 3rd branchial arches. Completely excise to prevent recurrence. Path- along carotid sheath, crosses hypoglossal nerve to tonsillar fossa
- Congenital midline cervical clefts- failed fusion of the 2nd branchial arches. Thin, red tissue in midline, excess superior skin, blind sinus tract, subcutaneous cord. Limits neck movement. Also have retrognathia, clefting of lip & mandible
- Adenoid cystic carcinoma of hard/soft palate- slow growing, spreads along palatine branches of maxillary division of trigeminal nerve
- Bilateral choanal atresia- paradoxical cyanosis (relieved by crying) in obligate nose breathers. Cannot pass catheter from nose into nasopharynx. Dx- CT- narrow posterior nasal cavity, medial displacement of lateral nasal wall & pterygoid plates, large vomer. Can have CHARGE (coloboma, heart defects, choanal atresia, retarded growth, genital hypoplasia, ear abnormalities)
- Lymphatic malformation- aka cystic hygroma. Soft, subcutaneous mass, respiratory distress if large
- Congenital subglottic stenosis- respiratory distress from narrow subglottic airway. Membranous or cartilaginous
- Benign masseteric hypertrophy- bilateral or unilateral. Enlarged masseter & temporalis muscles. Rx- muscle relaxants, anxiolytics, antiepileptic drugs, botox, resection of masseter, bone contouring for cosmesis
- Unilateral condylar hyperplasia- large mandibular condyle. Can have facial enlargement, deviation of mandible toward unaffected side, class III occlusion same side, crossbite on opposite side. Rx- condylar resection
- Condylar dislocation- Unilateral in hypermobile or stretched TMJ, happens suddenly, painful, class III occlusion. Rx- condylar reduction with muscle relaxants or surgery- eminectomy, eminoplasty
- Subcondylar fracture- lateral pterygoid muscle pulls proximal fragment anterior
- Maxillary canine- landmark for infraorbital foramen block
- Retromolar fossa- location for buccal nerve block to central cheek
- Lower lip lesion block- intraoral block of mental nerve
- Infraorbital block- upper lip & nasal sidewall
- Nasal palatine block- external nose
- Sphenopalatine block- internal nose & palate
- Glioma- encephalocele that does not connect intracranially. Red, firm, noncompressible, lesions at nose root with cutaneous telangiectasia. Won't transilluminate or pulsate

- Ranula- mucocele in floor of mouth. From sublingual or submandibular gland duct obstruction. Unilateral area of fluctuance, tinted blue or white. Rx- marsupialization or excision of gland
- Torus- slow-growing, hard mass of palate or mandible. Rx- excision if symptomatic
- Cutis aplasia of the scalp- absence of epidermis, dermis, soft tissue. Rx- small defect- antibiotic ointment, larger defect- STSG, flap

22. Head & Neck Tumors

- Saliva- parotid gland- serous, submandibular- serous & 10% mucous. Submandibular gland produces most of saliva if unstimulated, but parotid gland produces most if stimulated
- Sialocele- leak at parotid duct repair or injury. Rx- compression, aspiration, anticholinergic medications (↓ salivary flow)
- MC childhood parotid tumor- hemangioma
- Mucoepidermoid carcinoma- MC malignancy of parotid gland. Path- mucus & epithelial cells
- Adenoid cystic carcinoma- MC malignancy of minor salivary glands. Path- cribiform (Swiss cheese), tubular or solid
- Pleomorphic adenoma- aka benign mixed tumor- MC salivary gland benign neoplasm. Path- epithelial & connective tissue
- Warthin tumor- aka papillary cystadenoma lymphomatosum. Benign, slow-growing, painless, older men, bilateral. Path- papillary cysts, mucus, lymphoid tissue. Rx- superficial parotidectomy. Can recur
- Salivary malignancy presentation- facial weakness, painful parotid mass
- Salivary glands with highest incidence of neoplasm- major- parotid. Minor- palatal salivary tissue
- Merkel cell tumor- highly aggressive neuroendocrine tumors. Rx- WLE & SLNB +XRT
- Final salivary malignancy pathology with microscopic residual disease Rx- XRT. Gross residual disease Rx- reexcision
- Oropharyngeal tumors must be biopsied. Benign- resect based on symptoms
- Osteoradionecrosis of mandible- due to head & neck XRT. Hypoxia, hypovascularity, hypocellularity, impaired collagen synthesis causes exposed bone that does not heal in 3 months. Rx- debridement, antibiotics, HBO, reconstruction
- Ameloblastoma- benign mandible tumor. Xray- multilocular radiolucent lesion (soap bubble), by an impacted molar. Path- palisading odontogenic cells. Rx- segmental mandibular resection & reconstruction
- Bisphosphonate SE- osteonecrosis of mandible, orocutaneous fistula
- Radicular cyst- MC jaw cyst. Apex of nonviable erupted tooth
- Dentigerous cyst- degenerated enamel of unerupted tooth
- Gingival cyst- infant with soft alveolar ridge mass
- Oral cancer staging:

33

[handwritten left margin: R smoker]

[handwritten right margin: myoepithl both]

[handwritten bottom: Parotid 80% benign / minor salivary gland 80% malignant]

- - T1- ≤ 2cm, T2- 2-4cm, T3- > 4cm, T4- invading
  - N1- 1 ipsilateral node < 3cm, N2a- 1 ipsilateral node 3-6cm, N2b- multiple ipsilateral nodes, N2c- bilateral nodes ≤ 6cm, N3- any nodes > 6cm
- Oropharynx drains to level II nodes first
- Nasopharyngeal cancer associated with Epstein-Barr virus
- Angiosarcoma- 70+ years of age. M:F 2:1. Half in head & neck. Appearance is bruise-like or nodules that bleed easily. Poor prognosis. Rx- WLE, reconstruction +/- XRT
- Lip cancer Rx- XRT for <2cm tumor, >1/3 lip, commissure involvement, recurrent cancers, poor surgical candidates
- Neurofibromatosis 1- AD. Skeletal dysplasia (no greater wing of the sphenoid), macrocephaly, neurofibromas. 3 subtypes- localized, plexiform, diffuse. NF2 tumors are confined to CNS & similar to schwannomas
- Klippel-Trénaunay syndrome- capillary-lymphatic-venous malformation, hypertrophy of extremities & thorax of one side of body. Head & neck are normal. Skin is red with hemolymphatic vesicles. Embryonal lateral vein of Servelle present in lower extremity
- Parkes-Weber syndrome- overgrowth of extremity, microscopic arteriovenous fistulas. Head & neck are normal
- Sjrogren syndrome- xerostomia & keratoconjunctivitis sicca. Autoimmune destruction of salivary & lacrimal glands. Dx- biopsy of salivary gland. Lab- RF, ANA, SS-A, SS-B
- Nevoid Basal Cell Carcinoma Syndrome- aka Gorlin syndrome. AD. Criteria-
  - >2 BCC or 1 in patient <20 years old
  - odontogenic keratocysts of the mandible
  - >3 palmar or plantar pits
  - bilamellar calcification of falx cerebri
  - bifid, fused, splayed ribs
  - 1st degree relative with NBCCS
- Submental artery island flap- facial artery branch. Up to 7×18cm. Unreliable if a lot of neck dissection
- Karapandzic flap- circumoral incisions, mobilize orbicularis oris muscle, preserve lip nerves & vascular supply (superior & inferior labial arteries). Maintains continuous circle muscle & oral competence. SE- microstomia
- Lip defect Rx
  - primary closure- 1/3-1/2 lip width
  - Estlander flap- full-thickness transposition flap from opposite lip, used for <2/3 lip width, oral commissure defects
  - Abbé flap- transposition flap from opposite lip, central defects, remains pedicled for weeks
  - radial forearm free flap- total lower lip defects
  - facial artery musculomucosal flap- pedicled buccal mucosa & buccinator muscle flap, vermillion reconstruction
- Fibula osteocutaneous free flap- best flap for anterior mandible, especially with XRT. Skin paddle based on peroneal artery

- perforators. Do not use if blood supply to lower extremity is compromised, i.e. PAD
- Free rectus abdominis flap + iliac crest bone graft- reconstruction of maxillary defects
- Total laryngopharyngectomy reconstruction- free jejunum flap- restores pharyngeal continuity. Complications- thrombosis, flap loss, salivary fistula, stricture. Rx- debridement & repeat free flap reconstruction. Fistula Rx- NPO, wound care
- Upper medial cheek reconstruction- local skin is best. Example- cervicofacial flap. Close tension-free to avoid lower eyelid issues
- Radial forearm flap- radial artery + vena comitans. Cephalic vein can also be harvested to assist with venous outflow. Good for hemiglossectomy defect
- Latissimus & rectus flap- total glossectomy defect
- Scapular flap- circumflex scapular artery. Extend pedicle by including subscapular artery & vein. Chimeric flap- lat dorsi & serratus anterior muscles. Location precludes simultaneous resection & flap harvest
- Congenital midline nasal mass- DDx- dermoid cyst, encephalocele, glioma. Dx- imaging. Dermoid cyst- MC, may communicate intracranially. Encephalocele- protrusion of brain through skull defect, covered by the dura. Glioma- glial neural tissue not covered by dura
- Nasopharyngeal angiofibroma- benign, invasive vascular tumor in adolescent males. S/S- nasal obstruction, epistaxis. Dx- don't biopsy due to bleeding. Rx- excision +/- pre-op embolization
- Tracheoesophageal puncture prosthesis- used for speech in circumferential defects of laryngopharyngeal unit. Speech better with ALT & radial forearm flap vs. jejunal free flaps. → wet speech
- Osseointegrated prostheses- dental crowns, facial prosthetics, BAHAs
- Almost all dental prostheses survive in nonirradiated free fibula flap
- Glossectomy defect- restoring sensibility is very important
- ALT to floor of mouth- lateral femoral cutaneous nerve to lingual nerve anastomosis
- If no external carotid, use transverse cervical artery for microvascular anastomosis
- Face transplant- functional & aesthetic outcome is good. Issues- immunosuppression SE, skin rejection, nerve regeneration, donor legislation, public acceptance
- Skin- most antigenic tissue > muscle > bone > cartilage, tendon, vessels

23. Eye/ Eyelid/ Eyelid Reconstruction

- Anterior lamella- skin, orbicularis oculi. Middle lamella -orbital septum. Posterior lamella- tarsus muscle, lower lid retractors, conjunctiva
- Eyelid layers- conjunctiva, Mueller muscle, levator muscle, orbital fat, orbital septum, retro-orbicularis oculi fat, orbicularis oculi muscle, skin

- Medial orbital wall- mostly orbital plate of ethmoid bone, also lacrimal, palatine & lesser wing of the sphenoid bone
- Orbital floor- maxilla medial, zygoma anterior
- Superior orbital fissure- oculomotor, trochlear, abducens, lacrimal, frontal, nasociliary nerves; sympathetic branches; superior & inferior ophthalmic veins; orbital branch of middle meningeal artery; recurrent branch of lacrimal artery
- Optic canal- optic nerve & ophthalmic artery
- Inferior orbital fissure- infraorbital & zygomatic nerves
- Orbitomalar ligament attaches orbicularis to orbital rim, separating the lower eyelid from the face
- Inferior rectus entrapment with orbital floor fracture- downward rotation of the eye *(sclera trap door)*
- Inferior oblique muscle- CNIII- up & out rotation of eye
- Superior oblique- CNIV- down & out rotation of eye
- Superior rectus- CNIII- upward rotation of eye
- Inferior oblique muscle- between medial & central fat compartment
- Supratrochlear nerve- within corrugator muscle. Innervates central forehead skin
- Zygomaticofacial nerve- lateral fat pad of lower eyelid
- Trigeminal nerve- face sensation
- Infraorbital nerve- lower eyelid, cheek, upper lip
- Infratrochlear nerve- medial upper & lower eyelid
- Lacrimal nerve- upper eyelid
- Facial nerve- motor to face
- Palpebral fissure- opening between upper & lower eyelids
- Intercanthal distance= orbital fissure width
- Common canaliculus enters lacrimal sac posterior to medial canthal tendon
- Levator palpebrae superioris- eyelid elevation
- Lockwood ligament- fascial thickening that supports globe, around inferior rectus oblique muscles to capsulopalpebral fascia
- Mild eyelid laxity Rx- orbicularis repositioning with tarsorrhaphy stitch at lateral limbus *(orbicularis sling)*
- Lower eyelid laxity Rx- lower eyelid blepharoplasty & lateral canthopexy *(snap back test)*
- Severe lower eyelid laxity Rx- lateral canthoplasty & cantholysis
- Epiblepharon- congenital excess skin & orbicular muscle at lower eyelid margin. Pushes cilia against globe. Eyelid margin & tarsus are normal *(Entropion → excise excess orbicularis)*
- Ptosis- 2mm-mild, 3mm-moderate, 4mm+- severe
- Blepharoptosis- acquired dehiscence of levator aponeurosis. High eyelid crease, excellent levator function. Rx- reanastomose dehisced levator to tarsus
- Senile ptosis- levator aponeurosis dehiscence. Elevation of the supratarsal crease. Rx-levator plication or advancement.
- Congenital ptosis- young patient with moderate/severe ptosis, absence of eyelid crease, poor levator function. If sudden onset, rule

(handwritten margin notes: orb. wall, apex; laxity = tear trough; LR VI, SO IV; medial canthal tendon inserts anterior & posterior to lacrimal sac; inserts @ whitnall tubercle)

> poor out cranial nerve III compression. Rx- frontalis suspension @ 3-4 years old

- Blepharophimosis- congenital ptosis
    o Type 1- epicanthal folds, horizontally shortened eyelids, severe ptosis
    o Type 2- telecanthus, no epicanthal folds, severe ptosis, no levator function, lid skin shortage *frontalis sling*
    o Type 3- no epicanthal folds, telecanthus, antimongoloid slant of the palpebral fissures, severe ptosis, hypertelorism, skin deficiencies
    o Rx- repair of epicanthal folds, correction of eyelid ptosis, levator resection, medial canthoplasty, fascial suspension techniques used in combination

levator sling

- Involutional ptosis- MC acquired eyelid ptosis. Levator aponeurosis stretching, downward positioning of tarsal plate. Good levator function, high crease, thin tissues.
- Traumatic ptosis- excision or debridement of levator muscle at prior surgery. Rx- frontalis suspension
- Traumatic aponeurotic ptosis- good levator function, elevated eyelid crease, visualization of the shadow of the iris with eyelid closure, levator aponeurosis detached from tarsal plate. Rx- reattachment of levator
- Botox-induced ptosis- toxin migrates through orbital septum, ↓ levator palpebrae superioris function
- Mechanical, myogenic, or neurogenic ptosis- shadow of iris cannot be visualized through eyelid
- Ptosis treatments
    o Fasanella-servat- mild ptosis, good levator
    o Mueller resection- mild ptosis, fair to good levator
    o Levator advancement- moderate ptosis, poor levator
    o Frontalis suspension- severe ptosis, poor levator
- Levator function exam- stabilize brow, measure excursion of upper eyelid margin from down gaze to up gaze. Upper limbus- 2mm below superior edge of iris, 2 mm above superior edge of pupil
- Levator- 12-15mm- excellent, 8-12mm- good, 5-7mm- fair, 2-4mm-poor
- Poor levator function (0-6 mm)- frontalis suspension. Moderate function (6-10 mm)-levator resection. Excellent function (> 10 mm)-aponeurotic surgery
- Fasanella-Servat procedure doesn't address excess eyelid skin
- Levator advancement- eyelid will elevate 1mm for every 3mm of advancement
- Blepharoplasty examination of excess upper eyelid skin, eyelid ptosis, compensated brow ptosis (patient uses frontalis to raise eyebrows- automatic raising of eyebrows on eyelid opening)
- MC lower bleph complication- malposition. Also-scar, over-resection, orbicularis paralysis, edema, hematoma
- Eyelid excess fat removal can lead to cadaveric appearance
- Retroseptal approach to lower lid blepharoplasty reduces fat only

- Preseptal approach to lower lid blepharoplasty modifies lid-cheek junction
- Correct lower eyelid tone by tightening the muscle & canthal tendon, repositioning fat over orbital rim
- Pinch blepharoplasty removes excess skin
- Upper eyelid fullness s/p bleph- could be descending lacrimal glands. Rx- resuspension (not excision) of glands
- Dry eye syndrome- ↓ tears, discomfort that may damage cornea. S/S- pain, dryness, blurry vision. Blepharoplasty can worsen, especially in women on hormone replacement therapy. Wait 6 months after laser vision correction before blepharoplasty
- Tear layers- Inner- precorneal, goblet cells. Middle- lacrimal glands, osmotic regulation & infection defense. Outer- meibomian glands, oil layer prevents evaporation
- Congenital tearing due to nasolacrimal duct issue. Rx- massage, drops x 1 year, then probe
- Chemosis- conjunctival swelling & irritation after blepharoplasty. Rx- drops or steroid drops
- Facial nerve injury results in brow ptosis
- Place gold weights in facial paralysis patient's eyelids to assist with closure
- Anophthalmia- absence of the eye
- Horner syndrome- ptosis, miosis, anhidrosis. Loss of superior cervical ganglion sympathetics
- Myasthenia gravis- ptosis exaggerated with fatigue
- Thyroid ophthalmopathy- proptosis, diplopia, puffy eyelids, injected conjunctivae, lag
- Eyelid defects
  - >75%- cheek advancement flap with nasal septal cartilage & lining
  - <50%- cantholysis, lateral canthotomy & primary closure or Hughes tarsoconjunctival flap
  - FTSG from contralateral upper eyelid can be used for partial-thickness defects. Cross-lid flap for full-thickness defect
- Hughes tarsoconjunctival flap- take flap from upper eyelid, leave 3mm of upper tarsus intact, advance remaining tarsus & conjunctiva to lower eyelid defect. Advance skin-muscle flap from lower eyelid for anterior coverage
- Ectropion
  - Involutional- horizontal laxity of the eyelid
  - Congenital or cicatricial- vertical shortening of the anterior lamella of the eyelid. Rx- palate/donor/ear spacer graft
  - Secondary to paralytic entropion- paralysis of the orbicularis oculi muscle causing loss of tone
  - Neoplasia pulling eyelid away
  - Exam findings- abnormal snap-back test & distraction
- Post-op cicatricial ectropion
  - Monitor 6-9 months, massage, eye drops. Operate if persists or vision compromised

[handwritten margin notes:] excise will not do dry eye

lagophthalmos to

- - Rare with preseptal transconjunctival approach, 25% subciliary approach
  - Due to scarring of posterior lamella & septum
- Burn cicatricial ectropion Rx- FTSG, lateral canthoplasty. Avoid with early excision & grafting
- Asian eyelid- lack of levator aponeurosis insertion into dermis, no supratarsal fold
- Hyphema- traumatic hemorrhage of anterior chamber of eye. Rx- acetazolamide, steroid eye drops   high risk Glaucoma
- Subconjunctival hemorrhage- extravasation of conjunctival capillaries
- Hertel exophthalmometer- measures distance between anterior border of globe & anterior point of orbital rim. Enophthalmos is <14 mm, exophthalmos is >18 mm
- Lacrimal puncta close during eyelid closure
- Nasolacrimal duct- drains into inferior meatus below the inferior concha
- Epiphora- accumulation of tears that flow onto cheek
- Jones I dye test- dye instilled into conjunctival sac. Q-tip placed under the inferior turbinate at inferior meatus. (+) dye flows through the lacrimal system, exits at inferior meatus, dye on Q-tip. (-) no dye recovered- obstruction of lacrimal system
- Jones II dye test- localizes level of obstruction. Irrigate punctum with saline. (+) dye in nose, diagnose partial obstruction. (-) no dye in nose. Dye exits other canaliculus-obstruction in lower system. Dye refluxes in same canaliculus- obstruction in upper system
- Chronic mucocele of lacrimal sac Rx- dacryocystorhinostomy
- Blepharochalasis- aka dermatopysis palpebrum. Developmental deficiency of elastic tissue in eyelids. Unknown cause. Noticed in early adulthood. S/S- episodes of painless eyelid edema, baggy, thin, wrinkled eyelid skin. Rx- excise redundant tissue if vision compromised
- Pachydermoperiostosis- aka idiopathic hypertrophic osteoarthropathy. Inherited condition with progressive enlargement of eyelids, hands, feet & toes. Conjunctiva covered with hypertrophic papillae, ptosis, visual obstruction
- Retrobulbar hematoma- can lose vision. S/S- severe globe pain, scintillating scotomas, hemianopsia, amaurosis fugax, eye drainage, vomiting, coughing. Associated with ASA use. Rx- lateral canthotomy, mannitol, carbonic anhydrase inhibitors
- Coloboma- congenital ocular defect of eyelid, iris, retina, choroid, or optic disk
- Enophthalmos after facial trauma- ↑ bony orbital volume due inadequate fracture reduction. Rx- bone grafting
- Rhabdomyosarcoma- MC childhood orbit cancer. Rapid growth. Rx- chemo & XRT
- Strabismus Rx- intermittent patch therapy to strengthen rectus muscles
- Apraclonidine – α-agonist used to treat partial LPS dysfunction. Corrects 1-3 mm of ptosis by activating Muller's muscle. Not useful in botox ptosis

- Blepharospasm- involuntary, frequent blinking. Rx- botox
- Marcus Gunn pupil- afferent pupillary defect caused by optic nerve lesion. Dx- swinging flashlight test- pupil constricts less (dilates) when swung from unaffected to affected eye
- Hering law- eyelids are equally innervated. Correcting one ptotic lid reveals opposite hidden ptosis
- Bell phenomenon- upward, outer movement of eye upon closing. Absence will ↑ risk of corneal ulcer after blepharoplasty

24. Ear Reconstruction

- Six branchial arches:
  - 4th gestational week
  - Auricle 1st & 2nd branchial arches that develops 6 hillocks

    - Anterior (1-3) hillocks- tragus, root of the helix, superior helix
    - Posterior (4-6) hillocks- posterior helix, antihelix, antitragus, lobule
  - Meckel's cartilage- 1st arch. Malleus & incus
  - External acoustic meatus- 1st groove
  - Middle ear & eustachian tube- 1st pharyngeal pouch
  - Reichert's cartilage- 2nd branchial arch. Stapes
  - 2nd-4th branchial grooves- obliterate
- Posterior auricular artery- anterior ear, auricle
- Superficial temporal artery- auricle, triangular fossa
- Occipital artery- posterior ear
- Ear sensation
  - Great auricular- cervical plexus- from 6.5cm inferior to tragus along SCM- innervates lower half of ear
  - Auriculotemporal- mandibular branch of trigeminal nerve- runs with superficial temporal vessels- innervates tragus, anterior/superior ear, external auditory canal
  - Lesser occipital- cervical plexus- along posterior SCM- innervates posterior/superior ear
  - Auricular branch of vagus- travels along ear canal- innervates concha & posterior auditory canal
- Normal helical rim-to-head measurements- helical apex 10-12mm, midpoint 16-18mm, lobule 20-22mm
- Microtia
  - Hypoplastic spectrum from complete absence of the ear (anotia) to a small ear
  - Patients with isolated microtia have a mild form of hemifacial microsomia
  - US kidneys at birth to rule out anomalies
  - Rx- bone-conduction hearing aid by 1 year, autologous tissue @ 7 years old when enough costal cartilage, ear

development is complete & patient more compliant, ear canal construction in teenage years
- o Surgery in 2-3 stages- 1) create cartilage framework, place under vascularized tissue +/- tissue expander. 2) recreate posterior auricular crease, tragus, lobule
- o Continuous closed suction drainage for 5 days post-op. Pressure dressings risk skin necrosis
- o Porous polyethylene is acceptable option. Silicone has ↑ incidence of extrusion & infection
- o External auditory meatus & internal ear derived differently, so internal ear is usually normal in microtia
- o Bilateral conductive hearing loss- bone-anchored hearing aids, middle ear reconstruction after ear construction is complete
- o Post-op hematoma presents as severe pain within first 24 hours
- Otoplasty
  - o Stenstrom technique- cartilage abrasion with partial-thickness scoring of anterior surface of antihelix causing cartilage to bend away from scored surface
  - o Furnas technique- placement of conchomastoid sutures
  - o Mustardé technique- (MC) recreates the antihelical fold with posterior horizontal mattress sutures from scapha cartilage to conchal cartilage
  - o Webster technique- fixation of helical tail to concha
  - o Luckett technique- excision of postauricular skin
  - o Adequately reduce the cavum conchae before placing sutures to prevent lobule prominence
  - o Complications- MC is recurrence. Also hematoma, epidermolysis, suture extrusions, dehiscence, hypertrophic scarring, overcorrection, infection, palpability, asymmetry, unnatural appearance. Otoplasty post-op chondritis- antibiotics, remove sutures, drain. If fails- I&D, repeat otoplasty months later
- Ear molding- effective in infants < 3 months to permanently improve ear position, shape. Custom molding affixed to ear for weeks to months. Ear pliability from maternal estrogen, ↑ hyaluronic acid
- Osseointegrated implants- cancer extirpation, poor local tissue, absence of lower ½ ear, salvage, high risk patients
- Ear deformities
  - o Absent antihelical fold Rx- plication of concha to fascia with permanent sutures, or remove posterior wedge from conchal cartilage
  - o Congenital lop ear Rx- thermoplastic splinting for 2 months
  - o Stahl syndrome- aka Spock's ear. Hereditary abnormal cartilaginous pleat from antihelix to helix. Usual superior crus is absent, scaphoid fossa is broad & flat. Rx- newborn- molding, older patients- excision & helical advancement
  - o Cryptotia- adherence of helix to temporal skin. Rx- release +/- skin graft, V-Y, tissue expander, Z-plasty. Often left with visible periauricular scar, color mismatch, contracture

[handwritten margin note: Cru combos - & Stenstrom]

41

- o Pixie ear- complication of facelift
- o Prominent ear- wide conchal-scaphal angle, ↑ auriculocephalic distance, loss of antihelical fold
- Ear burn reconstruction- bilateral conchal transposition flap, skin grafting. Less preferred- costochondral grafts under existing skin, osseointegrated prostheses, silastic prostheses with temporoparietal flap, retroauricular release & grafting
- Conchal transposition flap- minimal donor site morbidity, helps with wearing eyeglasses
- Anterior concha lesion excision involves removing conchal cartilage. Reconstruct with postauricular revolving door island flap- posterior skin island rotated into interior conchal defect & posterior defect closed primarily
- Reconstruct helix with rim or rotation advancement flaps
- Antia-Buch flap- local flap of helical rim, postauricular skin used to reconstruct the helical margin
- Total ear resurfacing with temporalis fascia flap
- Partial-thickness injury Rx- debridement, topical wound care until devitalized tissues demarcate. Later use rib cartilage graft, temporoparietal fascia flap, STSG
- Elderly costal cartilages are calcified & brittle, difficult to use for reconstruction
- Middle 1/3 ear injury- postauricular transposition skin flap based at edge of the hairline, flap width equals defect. Divide flap @ 10 days. STSG donor area
- Need intact perichondrium for growth of a reconstructed ear
- Avascular cartilage will warp & contract
- Microsurgical ear replantation- debridement, dissection of vessels with microscope, anastomosis on the posterior surface. MC complication- venous congestion. Rx- leeches
- Auricular chondritis Rx- urgent OR, cultures, antibiotics
- Othematoma- shearing of skin from cartilage. Treat early to prevent cauliflower ear. Rx- small incision evacuation, bolster dressing
- Chondrodermatitis nodularis helicis- unknown etiology, old men, trauma from sleeping. Cartilage inflammation → skin ulceration. Rx- excision, closure. ↑ recurrence. Mimics skin cancer

25. Facial Palsy/ Lips/ Cheeks

- Bell's Palsy:
  - o MC childhood facial nerve paralysis
  - o Ptosis of brow & forehead, upper eyelid retraction, lower lid ectropion (cannot close eye), ↓ blink, ↓ ability to close eye
  - o Dx- exclude other causes- trauma, stroke, tumor
  - o Associated with diabetes mellitus & pregnancy
  - o 85% begin recovery in 3 weeks. 15% take 3-6 months
  - o Observe 3 wks before doing any diagnostic studies (EMG)

42

- o Ocular symptom Rx- artificial tears, ointments, taping. Eyelid tarsorrhaphy not necessary
  - o Contralateral botox helps achieve symmetry
  - o Endoscopic forehead lift at 1-2 years once recovery seems unlikely
  - o Gold weight helps close the eye
  - o Canthoplasty tightens the tarsoorbicularis sling
- Synkinesis- orbicularis oculi contracture with orbicularis oris contracture after Bell's palsy (eye closes when eating). Rx- botox
- Facial nerve injury- complete or partial paralysis of facial musculature. Primary end-to-end repair is best, but nerve grafting can be done. Distal end can be stimulated for 3 days after injury, after which neurotransmitter stores are depleted
- Great auricular nerve injury- C2-3 branches. Superficially crosses SCM 6.5cm inferior to tragus. Sensation to ear & postauricular region. MC injured nerve in facelift. Results in ear numbness
- Unilateral facial paralysis Rx- cross-facial nerve grafting from unparalyzed side to paralyzed side using sural nerve. Length of elapsed time from paralysis to surgery determines success. Second stage- free tissue muscle transfer
- Hypoglossal-facial nerve anastomosis- get good facial tone, but ipsilateral synkinesis when chewing. Rx- botox *cm 5- hypoglinatri*
- Free-muscle transplantation- reconstruct long-standing facial paralysis. Less predictable symmetry than cross-facial nerve grafting
- Neurotized free muscle transfer- restores dynamic function to face using a cross-face nerve graft or hypoglossal nerve
- Free gracilis muscle transfer- allows smile in complete facial nerve paralysis patients. Thin, contractile, minimal donor site morbidity, long motor nerve. Attach muscle from zygoma or temporalis to orbicularis oris lateral to oral commissure (simulates zygomaticus major)
- Gillies- flip middle 1/3 of temporalis muscle over zygomatic arch. Disadvantage- zygomatic bulge, patient activates trigeminal nerve for static motor function
- Cervicofacial flap- transfers skin & subcutaneous tissues from preauricular & neck area to cheek. Anchor flap to zygoma to reduce tension on lower eyelid *Obicularis sling*
- Central upper lip excision- reconstruct with bilateral Karapandzic flaps & central Abbe flap for philtrum
- Karapandzic flaps- maintains orbicularis, oral competence. Defects <80% of upper lip *sensate & neurohzed*
- Estlander flap- upper lip switch flap. Reconstructs lateral or commissure defects
- Radial forearm flap- reconstructs total lower lip defects
- Webster-Bernard flap- advances cheek skin by removing bilateral Burrow triangles. Reconstruct central defects
- Dog bite to lip- try to replace avulsed piece of skin & bolster
- Parotid duct injury- explore & repair ASAP. Dx- cannulate Stensen duct intraorally, inject methylene blue. Rx- repair proximal & distal

(handwritten: component & bulky)

ends over a stent & leave in place for 2 wks. If undiagnosed, a sialocele develops

- Frey's syndrome- gustatory sweating after rhytidectomy or parotidectomy due to auriculotemporal nerve dysfunction. Pathways of auriculotemporal nerve were disrupted & regenerate incorrectly, results in parasympathetic innervation of sympathetics. Rx- botox, Alloderm
- Lyme disease- can cause facial paralysis. Rx- doxycycline

26. Maxillo-Facial

- Vertical buttresses- nasomaxillary, zygomaticomaxillary, pterygomaxillary, condyle, posterior mandibular ramus
- Horizontal buttresses- aka posterior buttresses- facial depth. Frontal, zygomatic, maxillary, mandibular. Mandibular arch- only structure that defines the horizontal buttress of the face
- SCALP- skin, subcutaneous tissue, aponeurotic layer (galea), loose areolar tissue, pericranium
- Galea- strength layer of scalp. Contiguous with frontalis, occipitalis, temporoparietal fascia
- Anterior ethmoidal nerve- nasal tip
- Infratrochlear & infraorbital nerve- nasal sidewalls & dorsum
- Lateral branch of pterygopalatine nerve- upper & middle turbinates
- Medial branch of pterygopalatine nerve- septum
- Nasopalatine nerve- maxillary incisor teeth, gingiva, palate
- Pediatric skull fracture- rule out dural laceration, if missed will have growing skull fracture
- Non-depressed anterior wall frontal sinus fracture Rx- antibiotics, no surgery
- Depressed anterior wall frontal sinus fracture Rx- surgery for contour. If frontonasal duct is injured→obliterate sinus
- Non-displaced posterior table fracture, no CSF drainage Rx- antibiotics, no surgery
- Non-displaced posterior table fracture, with CSF drainage Rx- monitor, >10 days do craniotomy, dural repair, sinus obliteration or cranialization
- Cranialization- removing posterior frontal sinus wall, blocking the nasofrontal duct with bone or flap (mucosa excluded from intracranial space). Frontal lobe fills space
- Ablation (exenteration)- removing anterior frontal sinus wall, skin collapses to posterior wall or dura. Significant deformity
- Obliteration- removing sinus mucosa by burring bony walls, blocking nasofrontal duct, filling sinus cavity with fat, muscle, bone, alloplasts
- CSF rhinorrhea- elevate HOB, lumbar CSF drain, surgery last resort
- Beta-2 transferrin level- most specific test for presence of CSF
- Cribriform plate- ethmoid bone, home to olfactory bulb & nerves. Tears cause anosmia, CSF rhinorrhea

(handwritten: will still "smell" ammonia, trigeminal nerve)

- Mucocele- expands, symptomatic if untreated. Rx- complete removal of all mucosa with burr, obliterate duct & sinus
- Posttraumatic carotid-cavernous fistula- Abnormal connection between ICA & cavernous sinus. Rare with craniofacial trauma, but frequent with basilar skull fractures. S/S- pulsatile proptosis, ocular erythema, chemosis, diplopia, headaches, vision loss. Dx & Rx- cerebral angiogram
- Children <2 years old can regenerate bone over large defects if dura intact   *membranous ossification*
- Bicoronal incision- multiple, NOE, or frontal sinus fractures
- Methylmethacrylate- low cost, good strength, availability, doesn't incorporate into bone, susceptible to infection, does not grow with children   *Exothermic*
- Hydroxyapatite for cranioplasty- defects <25cm. Do not use- XRT, pediatric population because it will not grow with skull
- 7 orbit bones- ethmoid, frontal, lacrimal, maxilla, palatine, greater & lesser wings of sphenoid   *superior lim of globe*
- Lateral orbital wall- zygoma & greater wing of the sphenoid
- Medial orbital wall- ethmoid & palatine
- Medial orbital wall fracture- dissection plane between medial orbital septum & Horner muscle, reduces injuries to Lockwood ligament
- Orbital floor fracture repair indications- absolute- >50% loss of orbital floor (enophthalmos, diplopia), entrapment. Relative- diplopia without evidence of entrapment
- Orbital roof fracture- can have carotid-cavernous fistula, bruit, blindness, pulsatile globe   *superior orbital fissure syndrome*
- Orbitozygomatic fracture- orbital dystopia, enophthalmos, malar flattening due to downward pull of muscles causing ↑ orbit volume
- Trapdoor fracture of orbital floor- causes oculocardiac reflex- bradycardia, nausea, syncope. MC entrapped muscles- inferior rectus & inferior oblique. Rx- surgery to prevent ischemia & fibrosis of entrapped contents
- Enophthalmos- palpebral fissure narrowed & supratarsal fold deepened. Etiology- displaced zygoma, medial or floor orbital blow- out, NOE fractures resulting in ↑ orbital volume
- Medial canthal tendon- band attached to medial orbital wall. If displaced laterally, telecanthus occurs   *@ posterior- lacrimal crest*
- Transnasal wires for medial canthus reconstruction- placed posterior & superior to posterior crest of bony lacrimal fossa
- Retrobulbar hematoma- pain, ↓ visual acuity, trauma, periorbital/lid hematoma, chemosis, proptosis, ↑ intraocular pressure, ophthalmoplegia. Rx- lateral canthotomy & cantholysis within 90 minutes or blindness occurs
- Oronasal hemorrhage Rx- immediate anterior & posterior nasal packing, then embolization, MMF
- Telecanthus- ↑ distance between medial canthi
- Strabismus- lateral & medial rectus muscle attachments to bony orbit are irregular
  - → *head tilt to correct orbital rotation*

45

- Hyphema- tearing of iris blood vessels results in blood in anterior chamber of eye. Can lead to glaucoma. Rx- ophthalmology consult, intraocular pressure measurement, slit-lamp exam
- Subconjunctival hemorrhage- conjunctiva stains with blood from nearby fracture
- Corneal abrasions Dx- slit-lamp exam with topical fluorescein
- Infraorbital nerve injury- numbness between lower eyelid & upper lip. Occurs with most orbital floor fractures. Will improve with time
- Traumatic optic neuropathy- visual loss, ↓ color perception, afferent pupillary defect. MC etiology- optic nerve shear
- Marcus Gunn pupil- lesion anterior to chiasm alters the afferent pupil light response. Light into affected side→no constriction on that side, but consensual response on the normal side. Light into normal side→constriction of both pupils. Then light back to the injured side→paradoxical dilatation
- Normal pupillary constriction to light- retina→afferent optic nerve→ pretectal nucleus & Edinger-Westphal nuclei→parasympathetic fibers of oculomotor nerve→sphincter pupillae
- Cheek laceration- rule out facial nerve & parotid duct injury. Rx- repair over stent. Ligate if it can't be repaired
- ZMC fracture Rx- realign zygomaticofrontal, zygomaticomaxillary, infraorbital rim, orbital floor if >2cm^2 defect. Sphenoid reduction is most important
- Septal hematoma- between septal mucoperichondrium & cartilage. Can lead to perforation, fibrosis, saddle nose deformity. Rx- incision over hematoma, evacuation, loose repair, quilting sutures, packing, antibiotics. If bilateral, drain unilaterally or with incisions at different levels
- NOE fracture classification
  - Type 1- large central fragment. Rx- reduce & plate
  - Type 2- comminuted central fragment, intact medial canthal tendon
  - Type 3- comminuted tendon insertion. Rx- transnasal canthopexy

27. Mandible

- MC facial fracture in kids- mandibular condyle
- MC facial fracture in adults- mandibular angle
- Mandible fractures- young males. Half are unilateral. 1/3 have multiple fractures
- Symphyseal or parasymphyseal fractures usually have 2nd fracture near angle
- Angle fracture- Foreshortening on fracture side, posterior open bite on other side
- Mandible fracture through inferior alveolar nerve causes lower lip paresthesia

- Condyle is growth center for mandible. Vertical growth. Kids will usually remodel without growth disturbance, but can result in unilateral or bilateral hypoplasia. Rx- closed reduction, MMF for short duration *2-4 weeks*
- Mandible condyle fracture- S/S- blood in external auditory canal. Rx- closed reduction. ORIF criteria- displacement into middle cranial fossa, cannot obtain adequate dental occlusion with closed reduction, lateral displacement, foreign body
- Bilateral subcondylar fractures- premature occlusion of molars, anterior open bite, loss of posterior facial height, facial swelling, pain. Lateral pterygoid muscle displaces condylar neck medial & anterior, causing temporalis & masseter muscles to shorten facial height
- Dentition numbering- Maxilla- right→left #1-16. Mandible- left→right #17-32
- Angle class I- normal occlusion. Mesial buccal cusp of upper 1st molar occludes in buccal groove of mandibular 1st molar
- Angle class II- mandibular dentition is distal to class I position
  - Class II, division 1- lingually inclined *⟩ Incisors*
  - Class II, division 2- labially inclined
- Angle class III- mandibular molar anterior to normal position with maxillary molar
- Adult excursion- 40-50mm. Lateral jaw excursion-10mm on each side
- MMF > 4 weeks can result in ankylosis, hard to treat
- MMF problems- airway problems, poor nutrition, weight loss, poor hygiene, speaking difficulties, insomnia, inconvenience, discomfort, work loss & stiffness
- Pediatric fractures are treated more conservatively due to mixed dentition, elasticity of craniofacial skeleton, bone remodeling. Prevents growth disturbance
- Arch bars not an option in kids. MMF with custom splint and drop wires with circummandibular wires or bone anchor screws, avoiding dentition. Remove titanium plates in 3 months
- ORIF allows early mobilization, better airway control, nutritional status, speech, hygiene, comfort, earlier return to work
- Champy's principles- miniplates along mandible tension lines at fracture site. Monocortical screws. Anterior to canines, need two miniplates due to genial & digastric muscles. Posterior to canines- one miniplate only
- Use locking reconstruction bone plate to ↓ postoperative malocclusion in a comminuted mandible fracture
- Muscles of mastication- mandibular division of trigeminal nerve
- Lateral pterygoid muscle- origin- greater wing of sphenoid, lateral pterygoid plate. Inserts- mandibular condyle & disc of TMJ. Action- depress, protrude, moves mandible from side to side
- Masseter muscle- origin- zygomatic arch. Insertion- mandibular angle, ramus, condyle. Action- closes jaw
- Medial pterygoid muscle- orgin- lateral pterygoid plate of sphenoid. Inserts- medial ramus. Action- closes jaw
- Temporalis muscle- origin- temporal fascia, fossa. Inserts- coronoid process, anterior ramus. Action- closes & retracts jaw

- Submandibular space- inferior to mylohyoid muscle, superior to hyoid bone. Includes submandibular gland, lymph nodes, facial vein & artery, hypoglossal nerve
- Infection of 2nd & 3rd mandibular molars into submandibular space. Infection of maxillary molars into buccal space. Infections of anterior mandibular teeth into sublingual space
- Retromandibular incision- safe & versatile exposure. Less injury to marginal mandibular, temporal, zygomatic branches of facial nerve
- *10%* 5% of isolated mandible fracture patients have a cervical spine injury
- MC mandibular fracture repair complication- infection. Rx- I&D, antibiotics, oral care, remove infected tooth, maintain rigid internal fixation
- Bisphosphonate-related osteonecrosis of jaw- Stage I Rx- observe. Stage III- exposed bone, pain, infection, pathologic fracture, fistula. Rx- segmental resection
- Osteoradionecrosis of mandible- exposed, irradiated bone, nonhealing for 3 months

> vascularized bone graft
> p excision

28. Nasal Reconstruction

- 9 subunits of nose- nasal dorsum, tip, columella, sidewalls, ala, soft triangles. If >1/2 of subunit, reconstruct whole subunit
- Nasal sidewall subunit reconstruction- <10mm- primary closure, second intention. 10-15mm- bilobed flap. >15 mm- paramedian forehead flap. If both dorsum & lateral wall- cheek advancement flap for lateral nasal skin & forehead flap for dorsum
- Nose innervation- trigeminal nerve
  - V1- ophthalmic division- infratrochlear nerve (sensation of bridge & upper lateral nose) & anterior ethmoidal nerve (sensation of skin, dorsum of lower nose, tip)
  - V2- maxillary nerve- infraorbital nerve (sensation of lower lateral skin) & nasopalatine nerve (nasal septum & anterior hard palate)

Sphenopalatine foramen to incisive foramen

- Nasolabial flap- defect of nasal tip, ala, lateral nose. Superiorly or inferiorly based. Inset at 2nd stage. Can combine with cartilage graft. Based on facial artery

foramen

- Paramedian forehead flap- nasal lobular defect. Based on supratrochlear artery & supraorbital vessel branches

rotundum

- Dorsal nasal flap- aka Reiger flap- lower nose defect <2cm and >1cm from alar rim. Based on ophthalmic branch of ICA & angular artery from facial branch of ECA
- Bilobe flap- defect <1.5cm of nasal tip or ala. Design- aka Zitelli modification- rotation of 90°, with 2nd flap placed on nasal dorsum or sidewall. Wide undermining in submuscular plane to ↓ tension
- Septal pivot flap- composite flap of mucosa & septal cartilage. Provides lining & support
- Bipedicle mucosal advancement flap- Provides lining of ala defect. Based on labial artery & vestibular blood supply

V3 - foramen ovale

- Turn-in flap- elevate skin & attach to defect edges for lining. Doesn't provide support
- Contralateral mucoperichondrial flap- based on anterior ethmoid artery. Used for nasal lining over septal cartilage graft
- Septum composite flap- subtotal nasal reconstruction. Uses residual septum based on superior labial artery *NB > 0.8cm from wound edge*
- Helical composite flap- alar rim, soft triangle, columella reconstruction. Max size 1x1.5cm. Appearance is white, blue, then red. Need good bed & no smoking *↑ surface area of wound bed = ↑ nutrient content*
- Hinged septal flap- flap of septal cartilage used to reconstitute height of distal dorsum & tip
- Hull graft- auricular concha cartilage graft used to augment dorsum after resection or for saddle nose deformity
- L-strut- bone graft that restores tip projection. From nasal bones to nasal spine
- Secondary procedures in nasal reconstruction done @ 3-4 weeks- timing of vascularity & wound tensile strength
- Cantilever cranial bone grafting- proximal dorsal nose support. Secured to radix or frontal bone with screws & plate
- Bone allograft is easiest donor for nasal bone reconstruction
- Mohs- high-risk lesions (morpheaform carcinoma, recurrent tumors, indistinct margins, cosmetically sensitive areas)
- Rhinophyma- acne rosacea. Almost all men, 50-60 years old, Caucasian. Enlargement of lower nose, prominent follicles, large sebaceous glands, lymphedema. Rarely →BCC. Rx- tangential shaving
- 80% of food flavor is olfactory. 10% of nasal surgery pts have ↓ olfaction
- Gustatory rhinorrhea- clear rhinorrhea when patient eats. Taste is normal. Nasal surgery complication

Malingering = can NOT smell Anosmia
"Trigeminal innervation"

29. Orthognathic/ TMJ/ Chin

- Cephalogram- x-ray to analyze facial symmetry
    - sella (S)- hypophyseal fossa
    - nasion (N)- nasal & frontal bone junction
    - Point A- innermost curvature from maxillary anterior nasal spine to alveolar process
    - SNA angle- maxillary position in relation to skull base
    - Point B- innermost curvature from chin to alveolar process
    - SNB angle- mandibular relationship to skull base
    - Pogonion- most anterior chin point
    - SNPg angle- degree of chin prominence relative to cranial base
    - Porion- superior external auditory meatus
    - Orbitale- inferior point of orbital rim
    - Frankfort horizontal line- joins porion & orbitale

Ear to eye line

49

- Interorbital distance- distance between medial walls of orbit. Usually the dacryon (junction of anterior border of lacrimal bone & frontal bone. Normal- 25mm in women, 28mm in men
- Prognathism- projecting mandible. ↑ SNB angle
- Maxillary deficiency- inadequate upper incisal show. Rx- maxillary osteotomy with vertical lengthening
- Maxillary advancement for midface hypoplasia due to CL/P can cause VPI
- Superior repositioning of maxilla- SE- ↑ alar base width, cephalic rotation & ↑ projection of nasal tip, ↓ nasolabial angle, short, flat upper lip
- Bilateral sagittal split osteotomy MC SE- paresthesia of lower lip from stretching inferior alveolar nerve. Will improve
- Symmetric expansion of maxillary halves- osteotomies of anterior & lateral antral walls, pterygoid plates, midpalatal suture, nasal septum. Do not include lateral nasal walls
- Le Fort III advancement in kids- recurrence & reoperation common. Definitive orthognathic surgery at completion of skeletal growth
- Distraction osteogenesis of mandible phases
    o Latency- time right after placement of device. 1-7 days. No movement
    o Activation- distraction 1 mm/day
    o Consolidation- device in place but not active. 2x activation phase
- Distraction osteogenesis- large movement because of gradual stretching of soft tissue envelope. External device advantages- ability to mold bony regenerate, adjust dental relationships, longer length of distraction, ease of placement. External device disadvantages- facial scars, ↑ distance from distractor to bone surface. CL/CP scarring is an indication for distraction to gradually stretch scars
- Reconstruct deficient mandible in kids- cortical bone from iliac crest, calvaria, rib, radius, or fibula. Leave cartilage on end of rib to allow growth, but can overgrow- asymmetry, malocclusion
- Combined osteotomies of mandible & chin brings mandibular dental midline & bony chin midline to midsagittal line
- Retrognathia- ↓ SNB angle, normal SNA angle
- Lower lip ptosis- occurs when mentalis muscle not reattached to mandible during genioplasty. Lower dental show, drooling
- Mentalis muscle innervation- marginal mandibular branch of facial nerve
- Buccinator & orbicularis oris innervation- buccal branch of facial nerve
- Inferior alveolar nerve injury- occurs with bilateral sagittal split osteotomy or genioplasty. S/S- paresthesia of lower lip, drooling
- Descending palatine artery- IMA branch within palatine bone. Injury common with Le Fort I osteotomy, but will not cause necrosis
- Hemorrhage in orthognathic surgery- MC due to maxillary osteotomies- greater palatine vessels, maxillary artery, pterygoid plexus. Mandible osteotomies- inferior alveolar artery, facial artery, retromandibular vein, pterygoid venous vein

50

- TMJ disorders- ankylosis, arthritis, trauma, dislocation, congenital & developmental anomalies, neoplasms
- MC cause of TMJ ankylosis- trauma
- Clicking jaw- anterior subluxation of articular disk due to attenuated or ruptured posterior attachments
- Acute anterior dislocation of TMJ- masseter & temporalis muscles elevate mandible before lateral pterygoid muscle relaxes, therefore condyle pulled anterior out of temporal fossa. Unilateral or bilateral. Rx- closed reduction- down & posterior movement
- Eminoplasty- confines condyle to glenoid fossa by reducing or removing articular eminence allowing spontaneous reduction. Indication- symptomatic open locking of mandible. Rx- intracapsular disk repositioning, discectomy, or interpositional temporalis fascia flap
- RA- tenderness, swelling, ↓ TMJ motion. Condyle erosion leads to retrognathism & anterior open bite
- Bruxism- teeth grinding, dental wear, myofascial pain, TMJ derangement
- Condylar hyperplasia- unilateral, painless overgrowth with chin deviation *lower & upper extremity*
- Pfeiffer syndrome with airway obstruction Rx- midface advancement *anomalies* (Le Fort III osteotomy & advancement). Do not perform Le Fort I osteotomy until all maxillary teeth have erupted *lower Aperts*
- Apnea Rx- enlargement & ↓ collapse of airway by anterior displacement of soft tissues & muscles. Maxillary & mandibular advancement is usually >10mm
- Marfan syndrome- high-arched, narrow palate, constricted maxilla. Rx- Le Fort I osteotomy & palatal expansion
- Tooth layers
    - dentin- below enamel, yellow substance protects tooth pulp
    - crown- visible 1/3 of tooth enamel, dentin, some pulp)
    - root- 2/3 of tooth in bone (cementum, dentin, pulp chamber)
- Dental factures
    - Dx- xray
    - deep- extends to dentin. Cold & air sensitivity. Infection risk. Rx- cap tooth, xray at 3 months to see if pulp died
    - pulp injury- Rx- prosthetic or root canal
    - alveolar bone fracture- unstable teeth. Rx- arch bar
- Tooth show at rest- 2mm of maxillary incisors. Gummy appearance- more show of upper dentition. Can be caused by maxilla vertical excess
- Periodontal ligament- anchors tooth. Enamel- outer protective layer of tooth. Dentine, enamel, cementum & pulp- major components of the tooth
- Mixed dentition- both deciduous & permanent teeth present @ 6-12 years old. Maxilla eruption order: 1st molar, central incisor, lateral incisor, 1st premolar, 2nd premolar, canine, 2nd molar, 3rd molar. Mandible eruption order: 1st molar, central incisor, lateral incisor, canine, 1st premolar, 2nd premolar, 2nd molar. No deciduous premolars
- Canine tooth root- 30mm. Longest root extending into maxilla

≥ 9 yrs of age ; Alveolar bu jmft before eruption (CP)

- Overbite- Angle class II malocclusion. Due to prognathic maxilla, retrognathic mandible, or both
- Overjet- horizontal relationship of maxillary & mandibular incisors
- Crossbite- reverse relationship of maxillary & mandibular teeth, sagittal or buccolingual
- Open bite- lack of vertical overlap of maxillary teeth over mandibular incisors
- Overbite- vertical overlap between maxillary & mandibular incisors
- Angle class III malocclusion- common after CP repair. Scarring slows maxillary growth. Rx- Le Fort I osteotomy or distraction osteogenesis after skeletal maturity
- Angle class III malocclusion from mandibular prognathism Rx- mandibular setback not maxillary advancement
- Periapical cyst- MC odontogenic cyst. Non-viable, infected tooth leads to pulp necrosis. Dx- radiolucent on xray
- Dentigerous cyst- 2nd MC odontogenic cyst. Asymptomatic, normal dental follicle around unerupted tooth
- Odontogenic keratocyst- 3rd MC odontogenic cyst. Variable presentation. Rapid growing, aggressive, high recurrence rates. Part of basal cell nevus syndrome
- Mucous retention cyst- aka mucocele. Pseudocyst from trauma to minor salivary glands in lips

[handwritten left margin: Compre? SNA SNB]

[handwritten left margin: Gorlin Syndrome]

[handwritten: Ameloblastoma - mandible > maxilla; neoplasm; unerupted teeth; bony deformity; "soap bubble" appearance]

30. Congenital Hand

- Congenital hand categories
    - I- failure of formation- longitudinal arrest (club hand)
    - II- failure of differentiation (syndactyly, synostoses, Poland syndrome)
    - III- duplication (polydactyly)
    - IV- overgrowth (macrodactyly, hemihypertrophy)
    - V- undergrowth (brachysyndactyly)
    - VI- constriction ring syndrome (any level)
    - VII- generalized skeletal deformaties (apert, TAR syndrome)
- Embryology- 2 weeks- limb buds not formed. 5 weeks- limb buds present. 8 weeks- digital separation. 7 weeks- fingernails
- Thumb hypoplasia
    - I- minor hypoplasia. Rx-none
    - II- absence of thenar muscles, web space narrowing, UCL insufficient. Rx- opponensplasty, web space deepening, UCL reconstruction
    - IIIA/B- musculoskeletal deficiencies, CMC joint instability. Rx- Huber transfer (transfer of hypothenar muscle to thenar area) vs. pollicization
    - IV- pouce flottant. Rx- pollicization
    - V- absent thumb. Rx- pollicization of the index finger @ 1 year

[handwritten left margin: IIIB; CMC joint unstable; pouce; pollicization]

Keep intact UCL

- Wassel thumb duplication →
  - Type II- duplicated distal phalanx. Rx- reconstruct RCL
  - Type IV duplicated middle & distal phalanx. Rx- preserve UCL for pinch, transfer APB from base of radial duplicate to base of ulnar duplicate
- Syndactyly
  - occurs at 5-8 weeks of gestation. 1/ 2000 births. Usually no syndromes
  - Complete or incomplete- distal to proximal webbing.
  - Complex or simple- bony involvement.
  - Border digit syndactyly (1st & 4th web spaces)- operate at 4-6 months. 2nd & 3rd web spaces released later.
  - Operate by 18 months of age. Z-plasty. Post-op long arm cast
- Great toe-to-thumb microsurgical reconstruction is appropriate when most of the first metacarpal is present
- Baby with absent thumb- evaluate for hematopoietic abnormalities
- Kirner deformity- progressive palmar or radial curvature of the distal phalanx of small finger. Preadolescence. Frostbite *Clinodactyly (delta phalanx)*
- Symphalangism- congenital stiffness of PIPJ. Failure of differentiation. Absent flexion creases. Multiple digits
- Camptodactyly- flexion deformity of PIPJ within 1st year of life. Failure of differentiation. Rx- none unless severe- release of abnormal lumbricals, FDS, collateral ligaments
- Clinodactyly- delta phalanx, excessive radial/ulnar deviation of digit. Can be inherited. Surgery if severe
- Symbrachydactyly- short digits with syndactyly
- Macrodactyly- Rx- debulking, epiphysiodesis at the DIP, PIP, MCP joints when fingers are adult length. Amputate if painful or massive. Do not correct webspace
- Ectrodactyly- partial or total absence of fingers. Central hand deficiency *Cleft hand*
- Cleft hand deformity- AD. Rx- Snow-Littler procedure- palmar-based flap & index ray to close cleft & make first web space
- Holt-Oram syndrome- AD. Cardiac defects, arm anomalies, clavicular hypoplasia
- Fanconi anemia- AD. Radial longitudinal deficiency & pancytopenia. Dx- mitomycin C. Poor prognosis
- Nager syndrome- AR. Radial deficiency & craniofacial abnormalities
- Apical ectodermal ridge- defines the growth of limb during embryologic development. If removed the limb would be short
- Maffucci syndrome- multiple enchondromas, venous & lymphatic anomalies *Multiple enchondromas + hemangioma*
- Cerebral palsy- thumb-in-palm deformity limits hand function. Rx- release spastic muscles & stabilize joint
- Radial club hand- partial or total absence of radial border of arm. Thumb hypoplasia to radius absence. Radial deviation of hand
- Complete absence of radius Rx- centralization of ulna & pollicization
- Phocomelia- hand or forearm attaches directly to humerus or trunk. Due to thalidomide during pregnancy

10 = CO cardiac defect

53

Ollier - multiple enchondromas

- Trigger- MC at thumb IPJ. Trigger thumb Rx- observation until surgery at 3 years
- Amniotic band syndrome- sporadic rupture of amnion. Tissue snares fetus. RF- prematurity, oligohydramnios, ↓ birth weight, young multigravida mothers
- Capitate seen earliest on x-rays *first two to ossify*
  1st to ossify *Scaphoid → pisiform*

31. Hand & Fingertip Amputations

- Hyponychium- junction of nail bed & fingertip skin. Contains polymorphonuclear leukocytes & lymphocytes. Prevents bacteria from invading the subungual region
- Perionychium- distal part of lateral nail fold where it attaches to nail *split nail deformity*
- Lunula- white arc that marks the distal germinal matrix
- Germinal matrix- most proximal part of nail bed under eponychium. Makes 90% of nail. Scarring→ nail abscence
- Sterile matrix- distal nail bed. Adds layer of cells to nail, maintains nail adherence. Scarring → nail deformity *early loss of adherence*
- Nail growth- 0.1mm/day. 100 days to resume normal appearance after injury
- 50% of nail bed injuries have distal phalanx fractures
- 80-95% distal phalanx fracture patients have nail bed laceration
- Reconstruction of sterile nail bed- resect scar, split-thickness nail bed grafting
- Reconstruction germinal nail bed- full-thickness graft from 1st, 2nd toes or spare parts in multidigit injuries
- Synechia of nail bed- eponychial fold adheres to nail bed due to scar. Rx- resect scar, graft from another finger or toe
- Hook fingernail- lose nail support after fingertip trauma repair with tension. Nail curves palmar. Rx- remove nail plate & redundant nail bed that projects over fingertip, V-Y advancement flap
- Split nail deformity- due to injury, scar. Rx- excision, primary repair vs. full-thickness matrix grafting
- Pincer-nail syndrome- curving constriction of distal nail that causes pain. Etiology- psoriasis, ill-fitting shoes, developmental anomalies, allergic reaction, underlying epidermoid cyst, subungual exostosis, osteoarthritis. Rx- dermal & collagen matrix graft reelevates the edges *Dorsal or volar oblique*
- Treat reattached amputated fingertip eschar by secondary intention. Larger defects- STSG have ↓ sensation, local flaps- bilateral V-Y (Kutler), volar advancement (Atasoy/Tranquilli-Leali)
- Atasoy-Kleinert flap- V-Y advancement flap of volar pulp tissue useful for transverse, oblique, dorsal fingertip injuries. Primarily close donor site *Dorsal oblique*
- Flexor profundus tendon attaches to distal phalanx base. Loss- ↓ grip strength
- Thumb tip- needed for opposition & holding objects. Must have sensation & padding. Small defects (1 cm)- Moberg. Large defects-

up to 1.5 cm *sensate advancement flap*

54

- first dorsal metacarpal artery flap, Little flap (dorsoulnar long finger), or reverse radial artery flap
- Toe-to-thumb transfer- thumb reconstruction for injury at or around MCP joint
- Reverse posterior interosseous artery flap- pedicled fasciocutaneous flap. Reconstruct the dorsum of hand, 1st web space
- Distal aspect of the palm amputation- intrinsic muscles injured. ↓ finger abduction, adduction, MCP joint flexion, PIP & DIP joint extension, pinch
- Cross-finger flap- defects on volar aspect of adjacent digit. Flap sutured to recipient finger, receives FTSG
- Reverse cross-finger flap- defects on dorsum of adjacent digit. Flap sutured to recipient finger, receives. ~~FTSG~~ STSG
- Adipofascial turnover flaps- dorsal digital defects. Flap 2-4 mm wider than defect. Elevate flap proximal to distal from skin & paratenon, turn over, cover with STSG
- Toe pulp flap- improves bulk with sensate tissue. From lateral aspect 1st toe or medial aspect of 2nd toe. Supplied by 1st dorsal metatarsal artery of dorsalis pedis, deep peroneal nerve, palmar digital nerves
- First dorsal metacarpal artery flap- aka kite flap. Within first dorsal interosseous muscle fascia. Axial flap off radial artery branch after anatomic snuff box. Skin paddle- dorsal index finger. Veins- venae comitantes, superficial veins. Reaches dorsal & volar thumb
- Ligate ring finger radial digital artery when mobilizing a neurovascular island flap from the ulnar aspect of long finger for thumb reconstruction
- Moberg flap- volar thumb flap based on radial & ulnar neurovascular bundles. Covers 2cm^2. SE- IPJ contracture
- Thenar flap- young patients with index or long volar defect
- Degloving avulsion of ring finger- Class III injury. Rx- complete amputation
- Ray amputation- close space by suturing the deep intervolar plate ligaments
- Transposition of index finger to long finger done at metacarpal base. Better healing due to cancellous bone volume at metaphyseal flare
- Cannot repair FPL tendon if avulsed off musculotendinous junction. Rx- FPL resection. Still have good range of motion of thumb even if no IP joint flexion *Arthrodesis IP JOINT*
- Avulsion injury- large zone of injury of soft tissue. Rx- wide resection, vein grafts *Rotate or Reverse*
- Traumatic thumb amputation with EPL, FPL avulsion from muscle- reimplant & fuse IPJ *if able to complete muscular repair*
- High-pressure injection injury- damage caused by chemicals, which can travel through tendon sheaths. Rx- debridement ASAP, wound care, early mobilization
- Replantation
  - Finger indications- all healthy children injuries, thumb
  - Finger contraindications- single digits within zone II due to stiffness, when rehab delays return to work, single digits

55

- General contraindications- ischemia >6 hours, other life-threatening injuries, multi-level injury, crush or avulsion, extreme contamination, systemic illness, self-mutilation, psychosis
- Order- skeletal fixation, flexor tendons, extensor tendons, arteries, veins
- If equally-preserved multiple fingers, do group repair of similar parts
- Venous congestion after replantation- remove dressings & sutures, heparin, leeches, exploration. Cause is usually hematoma or bleeding
- Amputation proximal to wrist- establish blood supply <6 hours. Order- fasciotomies, bone fixation, repair artery, vein, nerve. Consider arterial shunting
- Thumb amputation- princeps pollicis artery, in anatomical snuff box, is repaired with vein graft from foot or forearm

Aeromonas prophylaxis

32. Dupuytren's/ Vascular Hand

- Dupuytren's
    - Myofibroblasts act on collagen to form cord
    - Proliferative stage- ↑ myofibroblasts. Involutional stage- myofibroblasts align. Residual stage- tissue becomes acellular with thick bands of collagen, ↓myofibroblasts
    - Spiral cord- pretendinous bands, spiral bands, lateral digital sheets, natatory ligaments & Grayson ligaments. Cord contracts & straightens, displacing neurovascular bundle centrally
    - Not involved- superficial & deep transverse ligaments, Cleland's ligament, Landsmeer's ligament
    - Fasciectomy indications- loss of 30° MCPJ extension, any loss of PIPJ extension, neurovascular compromise
    - MC- ring finger
    - PIPJ flexion contracture- often incomplete correction. Recurrent PIP joint disease- more extensive joint release, dermatofasciectomy with FTSG, arthrodesis
    - If PIPJ not released after cord excision, release checkrein ligaments
    - Diathesis- aggressive, earlier onset, rapid, bilateral, radial hand. Knuckle pads, plantar fascia involvement, Peyronie's disease
    - Nodules- plantar fibromatosis patients. Remain stable. Steroid shot if painful
- Arteriovenous fistula- from intravenous access. Blood flows rapidly from artery to vein. Dx- palpable thrill, duplex, technetium scan, MRA
- Hypothenar hammer syndrome- repetitive blunt trauma to hypothenar eminence causing ulnar artery thrombosis at Guyon canal, can embolize distally causing infarction. S/S- cold intolerance, pain, ulnar sensory dysfunction, mass, ulceration. Rx- vasodilators, ceasing

contract c (with) flexion contracture

56

activity, smoking cessation, sympathectomy, thrombolytics, aneurysm exclusion, ulnar artery ligation, or aneurysm excision & vascular reconstruction with vein

- Subungual hematoma- pressure between nail plate & bed, causing pain. Rx- drainage with heated sterile paper clip
- Buerger's disease- thromboangiitis obliterans. Fingertip gangrene in middle-aged smoker. Dx- arteriography- plaques in digital arteries. Rx- smoking cessation
- Thoracic outlet syndrome- compression of subclavian artery or brachial plexus (C8-T1). S/S- headaches, finger numbness, shoulder & chest pain with overhead arm lifting
- Volkmann ischemic contracture- due to untreated injury or fracture. Tsuge classification- based on susceptibility of muscles in forearm to ischemia & pressure. Deeper compartments are more susceptible. Holden classification- Type 1 caused by injuries proximal to injured forearm muscles. Type 2 caused by direct injuries
- Scleroderma- calcinosis, Raynaud's, esophageal dysphasia, sclerodactyly & telangiectasia (CREST syndrome), cold intolerance, ulcers, thin, shiny fingers
- Scleroderma tip ulceration Rx- debridement, silvadene, resection of exposed bone, antibiotics. Fails- amputation, digital sympathectomy
- Raynaud's phenomenon- progressive vasospastic condition. Middle-age women, ulcers, gangrene. Dx- cold stress vascular testing
- Amputation rate in diabetic patients with hand infections is 75-100%. Highest with CRF or kidney transplantation
- Squamous cell carcinoma- MC hand malignancy. 1-cm margins. Involves nail bed- distal phalanx amputation
- Collagenase injection- corrects flexion deformities of MCP joint, not PIP joint
- PIP joint contracture Rx- fasciectomy & volar plate release
- Long-term PIP joint flexion shortens neurovascular bundles. Careful with contracture release

33. Hand Fractures / Dislocations

- Salter-Harris fractures involve the physis
    - Type I- transphyseal
    - Type II- transphyseal, exit the metaphysis
    - Type III- transphyseal, exit the epiphysis & joint
    - Type IV- traverse both epiphysis & physis, exit metaphysis
    - Type V- crush injury of physis
- <8cm bone defect of hand- reconstruct with autologous bone graft (iliac crest corticocancellous graft) with rigid stabilization
- >8cm bone defect of hand- free vascularized bone flap (fibula)
- 1.5-13.5cm bone defect- distraction osteogenesis. Must have adequate bone stock for distractor pin placement
- Calcium phosphate cement- substrate for stable bone defects. Contraindicated in infected wounds

57

- Angulation deformities of little finger 40-70° have no functional impairment
- Index & long metacarpal neck fractures >10° need to be corrected due to lack of CMC compensation
- Metacarpal shaft fractures >30° in little finger, 20° in ring finger, any angulation in long & index fingers need to be corrected
- Jersey finger- avulsion of FDP tendon insertion. Type I- FDP retracts to palm. Rx- repair <2 weeks or tendon graft. Type II- held by A3 pulley, tendon retracts to PIP. Rx- repair within 3 months. Type III- large bone fragment held by A4 pulley. Rx- ORIF with mini-screws or wiring. Type 2 can convert to type 1
- PIPJ fracture/dislocation- stabilize with 30° of flexion & extension block splinting. After splinting, buddy tape for controlled extension. Other Rx options- ORIF, dynamic intradigital traction device with K-wires. Late presentation Rx- hemi-hamate arthroplasty
- Dorsal MCPJ dislocations- forced hyperextension. MC- index, little finger. Reduction blocked by flexor tendons & intrinsic muscles
- Bennett fracture- axial force through partially flexed metacarpal shaft. Volar lip fragment & metacarpal base. Main portion of thumb metacarpal is subluxed radial/ dorsal by pull of thumb extensors, APL, APB. Rx- CRPP or ORIF if failed CRPP
- Thumb MCP dislocation- dorsal. Disruption of volar plate, dorsal capsule, collateral ligaments. Reduce with gentle hyperextension of MCP joint, pressure on dorsal base of proximal phalanx. Can be inhibited by FPL & thenar muscles at metacarpal head
- Dorsal perilunate, transscaphoid, transulnar styloid fracture-dislocation. S/S- numbness, pain. Rx- closed reduction & splint ASAP, then to OR
- Displaced condylar fracture Rx- ORIF with screws or K-wire. CRPP more difficult. Nondisplaced condylar fracture Rx- splint, but x-ray frequently to monitor for displacement
- Elson test- central slip disruption of finger extensor. DIP extends with PIP flexion
- PIPJ collateral ligament injury Rx- buddy tape
- Mallet fracture Rx- hyperextension casting of DIP joint

34. Hand Nerves

- Classification of nerve injury:

Sunderland	Seddon	Expected recovery	Rate of recovery
I	Neuropraxia	Complete	Rapid
II	Axonotmesis	Complete	Slow
III		Variable	Slow
IV		None	No recovery
V	Neurotmesis	None	No recovery

58

- 5 levels of nerve injury: root, anterior branches of spinal nerves, trunk, cord, peripheral nerve
- Wrist blocks
  - sensation is blocked, movement is preserved
  - median nerve- innervates volar radial aspect of hand. Block between FCR & palmaris longus. Palmar cutaneous branch divides 5-7cm proximal to wrist crease- sensation to thenar eminence
  - ulnar nerve- innervates ulnar aspect of ring & little finger. Block between FCU & ulnar artery. Dorsal cutaneous branch- ulnar aspect of dorsum of hand. Block at ulnar styloid. Block at elbow posterior to medial epicondyle
  - radial nerve- innervates dorsal radial aspect of hand & first web space. Superficial radial nerve- block at radial styloid proximal to snuffbox
- Medial cord- medial pectoral nerve, medial brachial & antebrachial cutaneous nerves, median nerve, ulnar nerve. Can be injured at midclavicular line
- Lateral cord- lateral pectoral nerve, musculocutaneous nerve, median nerve
- Lateral antebrachial cutaneous nerve- sensory innervation of lateral arm
- Median antebrachial cutaneous nerve- sensory innervation of anterior/middle forearm to wrist
- Thenar nerve- can be injured in CTR
- Nerve transfer- use noncritical donor nerve to reinnervate a missing function
- Reinnervation of muscle should be done in <18 months
- Acute laceration Rx- primary end-to-end neurorrhaphy. Delayed or neuroma Rx- depends on gap size
- Open wound nerve injuries repaired early unless crush or soft-tissue injury. GSWs treated as closed because etiology is heat & shock- observe for 6 weeks, then EMG
- Sensory-only nerves repaired by epineurial approximation. Mixed nerves repaired with group fascicular repair
- Sural nerve- common nerve graft material. Formed off tibial nerve
- 1cm gap in digital nerve- polyglycolic acid conduit
- Synthetic nerve conduit- not effective in >2cm gaps, motor nerve defects
- Posterior interosseous nerve graft- good size match for digital nerve gaps. Little donor deficit, because it only provides wrist sensation
- Immediate mobilization of isolated digital nerve repairs is okay
- Nerve transfer is alternative to nerve graft when delayed or long distance
- Oberlin nerve transfer- restores elbow flexion in brachial plexus injury- FCU to musculocutaneous nerve
- C5-6 avulsion- external shoulder rotation by supraspinatus & infraspinatus muscles. Rx- transfer distal spinal accessory nerve to suprascapular nerve

- Transfer of radial nerve to axillary nerve improves deltoid & teres major innervation
- Cubital tunnel syndrome- numbness & tingling in ulnar nerve distribution, intrinsic weakness. Nerve runs posterior to medial epicondyle, between medial epicondyle & olecranon. Osborne band is roof of tunnel. Sites of compression- arcade of Struthers, medial intermuscular septum, anconeus epitrochlearis, FCU
- Ulnar nerve Guyon canal compression- intrinsic motor weakness with sensory sparing because lesion is distal to origin of dorsal cutaneous branch of ulnar nerve. Rx- release pisohamate & volar carpal ligaments. Zone I- proximal to nerve bifurcation. Zone II- area around deep motor branch to pisohamate ligament. Zone III- area around superficial branch
- Ulnar nerve recovery order: ulnar-sided flexion of wrist (FCU), abduction of small finger (ADM), flexion of MCPJ (FDM), abduct/adduct fingers (interosseous), adduction of thumb (AD) is last
- Ulnar nerve palsy- S/S- claw deformity, flexion of ring & little fingers, muscle wasting of hypothenar & first web space muscles. MCP hyperextension is prevented by dorsal pressure, EDC can extend middle & distal phalanges (Bouvier maneuver)- if not, then tendon transfer to dorsal apparatus. Proximal ulnar nerve lesion with segmental nerve loss will not regain intrinsic muscle function with nerve graft. ECRL transfer or Zancolli FDS lasso procedure can address ulnar claw posture of the fingers
- Ulnar nerve transection above elbow Rx- distal anterior interosseous nerve graft at level of pronator quadratus to deep motor branch of ulnar nerve (shortest course)
- Median nerve palsy- cannot oppose thumb or flex thumb at IPJ
- Anatomy at elbow- MAT medial to lateral. Median nerve, brachial artery, biceps tendon
- Median nerve in distal forearm- 20% motor, 80% sensory. Motor-thenar branch- abductor pollicis brevis, opponens pollicis, flexor pollicis brevis
- Median nerve exposed in forearm between FCR & PT
- FPB is distal to AbPB & OP and has contribution of ulnar nerve, so median nerve injury patients can still oppose thumb & little finger
- CTS EMG- ↑ median sensory & motor latency, fibrillations
- Median nerve compression sites- ligament of Struthers, lacertus fibrosus, transverse carpal ligament
- Abductor pollicis brevis- only intrinsic muscle innervated by only median nerve
- Radial nerve- innervates wrist extensors, ECRL, ECRB, thumb extensors, EPL, EPB, EDC. Rx- observe & therapy. Early should see improved function of ECRL, then ECRB, then finger & thumb extensors. If no function by 6 months, explore & repair nerve or tendon transfers- pronator teres to ECRB (wrist extension), FCU to EDC (finger extension), palmaris longus to EPL (thumb extension)
- Radial nerve palsy- cannot extend fingers, thumb, wrist or grasp objects. Rx- pronator teres to ECRB transfer restores wrist extension. Harvest PT from radius & weave into ECRB

most important for oppos fxn

60

- Radial nerve compression site- arcade of Frohse
- Radial nerve exposed in forearm between EDC & ECRB, arm between biceps & triceps
- Anterior interosseous syndrome- compression of median nerve in proximal forearm. Motor deficit only- impairs FPL & FDP of index finger +/- long finger, pronator quadratus. Classic pinch position- index DIP extends & PIP flexes while thumb IP joint hyperextends
- Radial tunnel syndrome- S/S- proximal forearm pain, no sensory deficit. Dx- pain with long finger extension
- Traumatic loss of musculocutaneous nerve- acute- primary repair. Chronic- restore elbow flexion with median +/- ulnar nerve fascicle transfer to brachialis or bicep feeding nerve
- Pronator syndrome- mixed sensory & motor deficit. S/S- median intrinsic & extrinsic motor weakness, forearm pain, radial palm, thumb, index, long, radial ring finger numbness, pronator muscle can be tender, firm, swollen
- Posterior interosseous nerve syndrome- compression of nerve after bifurcation above elbow. Only motor. S/S- radial drift of hand, wrist extension, lacks active extension of all fingers, radial sagittal band rupture leading to extensor tendon subluxation but can maintain extension of fingers if passively positioned
- Radiation-induced brachial plexopathy- radiation directed at chest, axilla, thoracic outlet, or neck. 1-5% incidence. MC- breast, lung cancer. S/S- sensory symptoms, swelling, arm weakness, shoulder, wrist or hand pain. EMG- myokymia
- Newborn with upper extremity palsy- Dx- EMG, then cervical myelography. Surgery if no biceps recovery @ 6 months. Poor prognosis if no biceps function @ 3 months. 90% recover spontaneously
- CRPS
    - S/S- constant, burning pain since injury, swelling, mottling, sensitive to touch, ↓ROM
    - Type I- no identifiable nerve involvement (aka- reflex sympathetic dystrophy)
    - Type II- identifiable nerve involvement (causalgia), MC in women & smokers
    - Dx- 3-phase bone scan
    - Rx- ROM exercises, avoid use, splinting, anticonvulsants, antidepressants, stellate ganglion blocks, autonomic nerve blocks, nerve stimulation. If fails- identify & correct the nerve injury (excise & implant into muscle)
- Compartment syndrome
    - Dx-clinical assessment or measure compartment pressure. Pain, ↓ sensation, weakness, worsened pain with passive muscle stretching, pain with passive finger adduction & abduction
    - Prophylactic fasciotomy- ischemia >4 hours. Curved incision from carpal tunnel, over volar forearm & straight incision over dorsal forearm. 4 incisions for intrinsic, thenar,

61

hypothenar muscles. Don't do digital fasciotomies unless really swollen

- Volkmann's contracture
  - o sequelae of compartment syndrome following a supracondylar fracture of the humerus
  - o contracted, functionless, pronated forearm, flexed wrist, clawed & insensate hand, hyperextended MCP joints, flexed PIP & DIP joints
  - o Rx- exploration & release of median & ulnar nerves, tendon lengthening procedure (muscle slide)
  - o deep flexor compartment muscles of forearm at greatest risk
  - o capillary endothelial damage at 3 hours, reversible muscle & nerve injury at 6 hours, permanent neuromuscular damage at 12 hours, leads to contracture
- Tourniquet intolerance- incompletely blocked musculocutaneous nerve. Rx- more local anesthetic in the sheath, coracobrachialis muscle, or at elbow
- EMG- abnormal conduction velocities- ↓ amplitude, ↓ velocity, ↑ latency. Low sensitivity but high specificity
- Tacrolimus- immune-modulating agent used in transplants. May improve nerve regeneration across a repair if started at the time of repair
- Blunt brachial plexus injury- Dx- MRI @ 4 & 16 wks. Acute Rx- nerve transfer, graft. Chronic Rx- tendon transfers if good donors & PROM, free muscle transfer
- Vibration desensitizes amputation stump neuroma

35. Hand Tendons

- Tendon reconstruction- must have good passive ROM, good soft tissue bed for tendon gliding, good patient compliance
- Tendon lacerations <60% do not require repair
- Optimal length of suture purchase in tendon repair- 0.7-1.0 cm
- Repaired tendon rupture- MC post-op day 7-10. Dx- MRI when flexion is contraindicated. Rx- re-repair within 2 weeks
- Late flexor injuries (>2 weeks) in zones I, III, IV, & V Rx- single-stage tendon grafting. Zone II Rx- pulley reconstruction with silicone rod then later tendon graft
- Ulnar nerve & artery are dorsal to FCU
- Zone 2 laceration & no FDP function, months later the FDP stump is in palm, tethered to lumbrical
- Only repair isolated FDP injury in young people that need dexterity
- Repair both FDP & FDS tendons- retain finger motion, ↑ power, ↓ PIPJ hyperextension, better FDP gliding
- Lumbrical-plus deformity- due to FDP tendon release. Rx- divide lumbrical muscle

- Boutonnière deformity- disruption of extensor tendon central slip at its insertion into middle phalanx base, extensor lag at PIPJ. Due to volar subluxation of lateral bands. Rx- splint PIPJ in extension & DIPJ free, if fails then surgery to reattach central slip or tenotomy, tendon grafting, or tendon transfer for lateral bands
- Swan-neck deformity- post-trauma or rheumatoid arthritis. PIPJ hyperextension, DIPJ flexion. Can be due to problem with DIP, PIP, or MCP joints resulting in volar plate laxity
- Jersey injury- DIPJ flexed. FDP avulsion. MC- ring finger. Type I- tendon retracts to palm, reinsert within a week. Type II- tendon retracts to PIPJ, reinsert within a few months. Type III- bony fragment stuck on A4 pulley, repair any time
- Scaphoid fracture malunion/spurs- can cause FPL tendon rupture
- A2 pulley cutting- tendon bowstrings away, ↑ moment arm, ↓ tendon excursion, ↑ power, ↓ efficiency
- Digital extension can be limited by- previous flexor tendon injuries (scar, volar plate contracture, collateral ligament contracture, poor skin at volar joint) & joint irregularity, arthrosis, or bony block
- Radial collateral ligament injury- forced ulnar deviation at MCPJ. Pinch causes pain & ulnar deviation
- Extensor indicis proprius- independent extensor tendon of index finger, overlaps EDC function. Can transfer to thumb
- ECRL/ECRB tendon transfer- whichever tendon isn't harvested powers wrist extension with ECU
- EPL tendon reconstruction- primary repair early or tendon transplantation late (PL interposition or EIP transfer)
- FPL rupture that can't be repaired- thumb IPJ fusion
- Restore thumb palmar abduction/opposition- transfer EIP to APB & anterior interosseous nerve to recurrent branch of median nerve
- FCU/FCR/FDS transfer to EDC reinstates finger extension in radial nerve palsy
- Palmaris longus tendon- middle of volar wrist, next to median nerve. Not powerful enough to provide finger extension, but can provide thumb extension
- Pronator teres better transfer for wrist extension than finger extension due to ↓ excursion
- Fowler central slip tenotomy- central slip inserts at middle phalanx base, acts on PIPJ. Tenotomy rebalances extensor mechanism so DIPJ can extend in chronic mallet finger
- Early mobilization of adult flexor tendon injuries- low force & moderate excursion
- Splint children with flexor tendon injuries for 4 weeks
- Juncturae tendinum- connect long, ring, small EDC
- Thumb opposition- palmar abduction, flexion, pronation
- Intersection syndrome- 2nd dorsal compartment tenosynovitis. S/S-pain & swelling of APL & EPB 4cm proximal to wrist. Seen in rowers, weightlifters. Rx- rest, NSAIDs, splinting, steroid shot. If fails, release 2nd dorsal compartment from wrist to swelling
- De Quervain disease- 1st dorsal compartment tenosynovitis. S/S-radial wrist pain worse with thumb movement, tender & swelling 1-

2cm proximal to radial styloid, + Finklestein test. 40-60 year old women. Rx- rest, NSAIDs, splinting, steroid shot. If that fails, release 1st dorsal compartment

- Extensor pollicis longus tenosynovitis- 3rd dorsal compartment- rare. Early surgery prevents tendon rupture. S/S- pain, swelling, tenderness, crepitus @ Lister's tubercle. Rx- 3rd dorsal compartment release, tendon transposition radial to Lister's tubercle
- EPL tendon rupture- 1% of distal radius fractures treated with closed reduction. Due to inflammatory synovitis in 3rd dorsal compartment & ischemia of EPL tendon. Dx- US. Rx- EIP tendon transfer

also for distal radius fracture dorsal approach

36. Hand Tumors

- Osteochondroma- cartilage-covered bone growth arising from bone surface. MC bone tumor in kids, single or multiple, spontaneous or trauma. AD in Bessel-Hagen syndrome or hereditary multiple exostoses). Occasional malignant transformation. Rx- wide resection & reconstruction
- Enchondroma- benign, cartilaginous lesion. MC bone tumor of hand. 1/3 of all arise in hand. MC in proximal phalanx. Dx- incidental xray finding, pathologic fracture. Rx- stabilize the fracture, followed by curettage, bone grafting & fixation. Can follow small ones with x-ray. Small percentage will recur

draw - multiple enchondromas

Maffucci syndrome- multiple enchondromas, hemangiomas. ↑ risk of chondrosarcoma
- Soft-tissue sarcoma- epithelioid sarcoma, synovial sarcoma, malignant fibrous histiocytoma. Rx- wide local excision
- Epithelioid sarcoma- pre-op XRT ↓ tumor size & recurrence. Chemo for high grade, >10 cm, lymph node involvement, or metastases. Rx- wide excision with negative margins
- Verrucous-type squamous cell carcinoma of fingernail- index, long, ring fingers. Due to HPV. Rx- Mohs superior to standard excision
- Glomus tumor- painful benign lesion arising from arteriovenous thermoregulatory glomus body. MC as solitary nail bed lesion. No mass visible. F:M 2:1. Dx- cold stimulation test. Rx- direct transungual or lateral subperiosteal resection
- Pyogenic granuloma- benign vascular tumor, unknown etiology, rapid growth, bleeds. Associated with pregnancy. Rx- shave removal & cauterization or surgical excision
- Merkel cell carcinoma- rare, aggressive skin cancer of neuroendocrine origin. Flesh-colored or bluish-red nodule on face, head, or neck. MC in elderly
- Neurilemoma- aka schwannoma. MC benign nerve tumor of upper extremity. Proliferation of Schwann cells on flexor surface of hand & forearm. Painless but with paresthesia or neurologic deficits. + Tinel sign. Mobile transversely but not longitudinally. Rx- shell out from nerve. Doesn't recur, occasional malignant transform

- Neurofibroma- benign nerve tumors arising from nerve fascicles. Difficult to excise & may need nerve reconstruction
- Ganglion- MC soft-tissue tumor of hand, age 20-40, F:M 3:1. Volar wrist ganglia from radiocarpal or scaphotrapezial joint; dorsal wrist ganglia from scapholunate ligament. Rx- surgical excision
- Mucous cyst- aka ganglion. Under eponychial fold, deforms germinal matrix *Remove osteophyte*
- Infantile digital fibromatosis- 5 months-6 years old. Broad-based mass on dorsal or lateral fingers. Path- intracytoplasmic inclusion bodies. Rx- wide excision +FTSG or local flap. Will recur if not totally excised
- Hand AVM- selective embolization of lesion
- Radial artery pseudoaneurysm- ligate if ulnar artery can perfuse hand. If not resect & repair with vein graft
- Lipoma- MC body tumor. Thenar eminence > dorsal or volar side of digits. F:M 2:1
- Epidermal cyst- M:F 2:1. Middle age. Distal phalanges of index or long
- Giant cell tumor of tendon sheath- aka- local nodular tenosynovitis, fibrous xanthoma. MC solid hand tumor, benign, brown, M=F, 4th-6th decade, MC in index & long, often recur
- Elevation & compression of brachial artery above the elbow for one minute in patients with neoplastic tumors. Do not exanguinate the arm due to possible dissemination

E Eschnuck

37. Wrist

- MC wrist fractures- distal radius > scaphoid > triquetrum > trapezium > lunate
- Distal radius fracture- >40 years, W>M due to osteoporosis. Fall on outstretched hand
- Most sensitive test for scaphoid fracture- MRI
- Scaphoid malunion Rx- interposition wedge bone graft if lateral intrascaphoid angle >45° (normal 30-40°)
- Proximal row carpectomy- regain most of grip strength & 50% ROM. No more pain. Need intact capitolunate surface
- Carpal tunnel view xray- hyperextended wrist showing carpal bone to carpal tunnel relationship, including hook of hamate, pisotriquetral joint, trapezium, pisiform & triquetrum
- Scapholunate separation results in flexion of scaphoid & dorsiflexion of lunate. Xray- ring sign due to scaphoid viewed end-on. ↑ scapholunate angle on lateral x-ray (>80°, normal 30-60°)
- Perilunate dislocation- MC carpal dislocation. Due to rupture of scapholunate & lunotriquetral ligaments *High energy injury*
- Wagner and Mayfield Progressive Perilunate Instability (PLI). 4 stages: PLI stage 1- mild isolated scapholunate dissociation. PLI stage 2- distal row & scaphoid progress dorsally, capitate separates from lunate. PLI stage 3- lunotriquetral ligaments separate. PLI stage

65

4- most severe, dislocated capitate dislodges lunate pushing it volar, creating lunate dislocation

- Scapholunate advanced collapse (SLAC wrist)- radioscaphoid, capitolunate & scaphocapitate arthritis. Capitate migrates between scaphoid & lunate. Rx- total wrist arthrodesis causes ↓ mobility, therefore limited wrist arthrodesis (scaphoidectomy & four-corner fusion) is preferred
- Degenerative arthritis of thumb- MC @ CMC joint of dominant hand. Dx- + grind test (crepitus with axial loading & rotation of metacarpal). 33% of post-menopausal women. Xrays- destruction of joint surface & space. Rx- rest, splint, NSAIDs, thenar strengthening. If fails then arthrodesis, trapezium hemiprosthesis, ligament reconstruction-tendon interposition arthroplasty, trapeziectomy. Trapezium excision & casting may be equivalent to soft-tissue spacer or ligament reconstruction. Arthrodesis limits mobility, silicone implants are inferior
- Eaton classification based on xray-
    - Stage I- normal or wide joint. Rx- splint, NSAIDs, trapezial hemi-resection or metacarpal osteotomy if symptomatic
    - Stage II- trapeziometacarpal (TM) joint narrowing. Rx- same as Stage I, but also CMC fusion if laborer
    - Stage III- TM joint narrowing, cystic or sclerotic changes of joint surface, subluxation of TM joint. Rx- trapeziectomy +/- ligament reconstruction/tendon interposition (LRTI)
    - Stage IV- TM & ST joints are destroyed. Rx- LRTI
- Laxity of volar anterior oblique (beak) ligament- first sign of basilar joint thumb arthritis
- Polyurethaneurea (Artelon)- biomaterial most appropriate for arthroplasty

38. Rheumatoid Hand

- Chronic, systemic inflammatory disorder that affects synovial joints
- 1% of US population. F:M 3:1, onset @ 25-50 years
- Dx- 4 of 7: morning stiffness >1 hr, arthritis of 3+ joints, hand arthritis, bilateral joint involvement, +serum RF, rheumatoid nodules, xray evidence of RA
- Anemia in 80%. ↑ ESR in 90%. +serum RF in 70%
- Joint fluid analysis- leukocyte count 2000-5000/mm^3 without crystals or bacteria
- Ulnar drift & pain on passive flexion Rx- MCPJ silicone prosthesis arthroplasty
- Tendon rupture- wear over bony prominence, synovitis, ischemia, painless, not immediately noticed. MC- ulnar-sided extensor tendons > EPL (cannot extend thumb IPJ). Rx- tendon grafts & transfers, remove bony prominences
- Trigger fingers in RA- due to intratendinous nodules & synovial inflammation. Rx- steroid injection then surgery. Do not divide A1

- pulley (prevents ulnar drift), flexor tenosynovectomy, removal of intratendinous nodules, resection of one slip of FDS
- Cannot extend extensor tendons- DDx- posterior interosseous nerve compression, extensor tendon rupture, MCPJ dislocation
- PIN entrapment in RA- elbow joint swelling leads to compression of PIN @ arcade of Frohse. Rx- steroid injection, surgery

note only

- Caput-ulnae syndrome- distal ulna dorsal dislocation from synovitis, ligament laxity & ECU tendon translocation. Risk of EDC rupture
- Swan-neck deformity- PIPJ hyperextension & DIPJ flexion. Four categories-
    - Type I- flexible PIPJ with any MCPJ position
        - Rx- figure-of-eight splint
    - Type II- limited PIPJ flexion with MCP extension (intrinsics tight)
        - figure-of-eight splint or intrinsic release
    - Type III- limited PIPJ flexion in all MCPJ positions (lateral bands)
        - Rx- translocation of lateral bands, PIPJ capsulectomy, collateral ligament release
    - Type IV- PIPJ destroyed
        - Rx- PIP joint arthrodesis or silicone arthroplasty
- Can also have deformity of wrist, PIPJ & DIPJ. Reconstruct from proximal to distal joints. If significant wrist pain, address that prior to MCPJ arthroplasty
- PIPJ arthroplasty- no change in ROM, ↓ pain, ↑ patient satisfaction

Treat proximal 1st

39. Microsurgery

- 5-25% of free flaps are reexplored for vessel compromise. Venous congestion > arterial issues. Most reexplorations occur within 48 hrs. Improved salvage based on timing of reexploration
- Microvascular thrombosis- MC within 12 hrs, often occurs intraoperatively. MC technical issues. Can be delayed up to 14 days postoperatively. S/S- purple color, brisk capillary refill, edema, oozing, hematoma. Rx- reexplore, leech salvage
- Monitor free flap perfusion- color, temperature, turgor, dopple. Use implantable doppler monitoring if buried flap
- Coupler- device for creating microvascular anastomoses. MC-venous. Place ends through ring & secure. Used end-to-end or end-to-side. Contraindicated- atherosclerotic calcification. Good for vessel-size mismatches
- Anastomosis patency- surgical precision, vessel size, blood flow, tension, anticoagulation
- No evidence of anticoagulation improving microvascular patency rates or free flap survival
- TPA- plasminogen→plasmin. Dissolves clot formed within flap
- Dextran & heparin- platelet inhibition, anticoagulation to improve free flap patency

→ *hypersensitivity*
depletes vWF

most venous side of flap

67

- Dextran- prevents clot formation, mild thrombolytic, not as effective as tPA. SE- ARDS (due to ↓ platelet aggregation, ↑ fibrin degradation, inhibiting alpha-2 plasmin, ↓ factor VII & von Willebrand factor, altering platelet function, volume expansion) & renal failure (do not use in CRF patients). Anaphylaxis possible
- Heparin irrigation- prepare vessels for anastomosis. Heparin can prevent but not dissolve clot
- Lidocaine & papaverine- used locally to dilate vessels
- Milrinone- systemic vasodilator that does not improve free flap patency
- Aspirin- prevents further clot formation, not thrombolytic, slow onset
- Aspirin should be used over dextran for flap anticoagulation due to SE
- Free flap procedure codes include- flap elevation, exposing donor vessels, flap transfer, exposing recipient vessels, anastomosis of 1 artery & 2 veins, microscope use, flap inset, donor site closure. Add-on free flap codes- vein grafts, neurorrhaphy, nerve grafts, STSG, complex closure of donor site, recipient site prep

40. Flaps

- Mathes and Nahai classification:
  - Type I- 1 vascular pedicle- gastrocnemius, rectus femoris, tensor fascia lata
  - Type II- 1 dominant & 1 minor pedicle- abductor digiti minimi, abductor hallucis, biceps femoris, flexor digitorum brevis, gracilis, peroneus longus, peroneus brevis, platysma, semitendinosus, soleus, sternocleidomastoid, temporalis, trapezius, vastus lateralis
  - Type III- 2 dominant pedicles- gluteus maximus, rectus abdominis, serratus anterior, semimembranosus
  - Type IV- multiple segmental pedicles- extensor digitorum longus, extensor hallucis longus, flexor digitorum longus, flexor hallucis longus, sartorius, tibialis anterior
  - Type V- 1 dominant & secondary segmental pedicles- pectoralis major, lat dorsi
- Prelaminated flap- recreates missing tissues at the donor site prior to flap transfer with skin, mucosa, cartilage, bone
- Delayed flap- divide some vasculature prior to final flap elevation to ↑ perfusion
- Freestyle flap- flap harvested using doppler signals, dissect pedicle. Unknown anatomy
- Prefabricated flap- transfer pedicle into ideal area for angiogenesis, then transfer somewhere else
- Tubularized flap- sew to itself creating a tube (ALT flap used for pharyngoesophageal reconstruction)

- Arterialized venous free flaps- thin fasciocutaneous flaps. Hand defects. Easy, no major artery sacrifice, venous congestion, difficult to monitor flap
- Juri flaps- frontal or frontoparietal defects. Parietal branch of superficial temporal artery. Delay the distal aspect prior to surgery
- Orticochea procedure- occiput defect. Can cover up to 30% scalp defect. Poor cosmesis due to hair orientation
- Free tissue transfer for total scalp defects. Ex- lat dorsi, radial forearm, ALT, parascapular flaps
- Superficial temporal fascia- superficial temporal artery
- Temporoparietal fascial flap- thin fascial free flap for reconstruction of injuries that cannot be covered with STSG- exposed tendons or joints. Supplied by superficial temporal artery
- Posterior interosseous flap- pedicled forearm flap off posterior interosseous artery. Covers elbow, antecubital fossa, proximal volar forearm defects. Dissect pedicle distally in forearm between ECU & EDM. Watch out for motor nerves *Radial & PIN*
- Lateral arm flap- posterior radial collateral artery. 12x6-cm flap. Major extremity vessels undisturbed
- Reverse lateral arm flap- supplied by radial recurrent artery *Henry Kim*
- Radial forearm flap- supplied by radial artery. Deep to brachioradialis muscle, then between brachioradialis & FCR. Skin perfused by septocutaneous perforators
- Radial forearm osteofasciocutaneous flap- harvest at radial aspect of radius between brachioradialis & pronator teres. Harvest up to 10 cm length, 40% of cross-sectional area. Superficial branch of radial nerve can be sacrificed
- Lateral arm flap- posterior radial collateral artery, branch of profunda brachial artery. Harvested from same extremity. Thin, pliable skin. +/- nerve, humerus, triceps tendon. Contoured for hand defects
- Medial arm flap- superior ulnar collateral artery. Many variations, so not a good flap
- Trapezius flap- dorsal scapular artery off subclavian artery. Superior trapezius- occipital artery. Middle trapezius- superficial cervical artery. Covers posterior neck wounds
- Latissimus dorsi muscle free flap- large scalp defects
- Paraspinous muscle, reverse latissimus dorsi flap- posterior intercostal artery
- Subscapular flap- circumflex scapular artery off scapular artery 4cm from axillary artery. Flap up to 25cm with primary closure. Chimeric flaps- bone, muscle, fascia, fat & skin. Serratus anterior muscle & fascia, latissimus dorsi muscle & fascia, scapular & parascapular fascia & skin, and scapular & rib bone. Useful for complex facial defects
- Iliac crest free flap- deep circumflex iliac artery off external iliac. Useful for maxilla & mandible reconstruction
- ALT flap- descending branch of lateral femoral circumflex artery off profunda femoris artery, located between vastus lateralis & rectus femoris. Large skin territory. No major vessel sacrifice. Try for septocutaneous perforators or harvest muscle cuff around

69

perforators. Vastus lateralis can be harvested with ALT flap to add bulk. Lateral femoral cutaneous nerve added for sensation. Useful for circumferential pharyngeal defects

- Rectus femoris flap- covers abdomen, groin, hip. Inserts into patella, so repair following harvest. ↓ 15° knee extension. Primarily close donor site
- Gluteal musculocutaneous flap- superior & inferior gluteal arteries off internal iliac. Can be a V-Y advancement flap
- Tensor fascia lata flap- ascending branch of lateral femoral circumflex artery
- S-GAP flap- superficial branch of gluteal artery serves fat & skin of the region. Allows preservation of donor site muscle with reliable skin & soft-tissue flap. 2-3 perforators arise from this vessel, with pedicle length of 3-8 cm
- Fibular free flap- reconstruction of large segmental bone defects. Must leave proximal & distal 6cm. +/- lateral skin paddle based on perforators through lateral intermuscular septum or muscle. Peroneal artery pedicle- next to FHL in deep posterior compartment. Include cuff of FHL to protect pedicle & add bulk. Expect post-op pain with walking. Complications- perineal & posterior tibial nerve injury, unstable ankle
- Gracilis muscle flap- ascending branch of medial femoral circumflex artery. Obturator nerve runs with vascular pedicle. Pedicle can be 6cm long, 2mm diameter. Between adductor longus & adductor brevis muscles. Sacrifice 2 minor vascular pedicles off SFA. No functional loss. Covers medial thigh & groin defects. Cannot rotate distally
- Gastrocnemius flap- medial & lateral sural arteries (popliteal branch). Covers complex knee wounds. +/-skin vs. STSG. Best coverage for distal knee wound is medial gastroc
- Sartorius flap- covers infected groin vascular graft. Origin- ASIS. Insertion- medial tibia. Type V muscle flap- segmental perforators of SFA. Proximal pedicle- 6cm from ASIS
- Soleus flap- branches of posterior tibial, popliteal & peroneal artery. Covers middle 1/3 of leg
- Lateral calcaneal flap- lateral calcaneal artery, branch of peroneal artery. Covers lateral malleolus. Other options- reverse sural or free tissue
- Medial plantar flap- medial plantar artery & nerve. Covers heel
- Rectus flap- for chest wall reconstruction it's pedicled on superior epigastric vessels. Can't us if IMA was used in CABG
- External oblique turnover muscle flap- covers large back defects. Upper flap supplied by 4th-11th intercostal arteries, lower supplied by deep circumflex iliac or iliolumbar artery
- Omental flap- gastroepiploic arteries. Passed through diaphragm or abdominal wall
- W-plasty- interdigitating triangular advancement flaps. Used for scar revisions over relaxed skin tension lines, convex or concave surfaces. ↓ contracture

- Fasciocutaneous muscle flap- fat of flap allows tendons and nerves to glide
- Dog ear after rotation flap- observe 2 months. Most resolve

41. Lower Extremity

- Gustilo classification of open fractures- severity of soft tissue & vascular injury
  - Type I- clean wound, <1cm, minimally comminuted bone
  - Type II- contaminated wound, >1cm, moderate comminuted bone
  - Type IIIA- highly contaminated wound, 1-10cm, severe comminuted bone
  - Type IIIB- highly contaminated wound, >10cm, severe comminuted bone
  - Type IIIC- major vascular injury compromising limb

  [handwritten: free flap coverage]

- Gustilo Type IIIB/C fractures need to be covered within 72 hours. Highest risk of infection & flap loss 3-90 days
- Open fracture sequence- external fixation, free muscle flap, bone graft (if needed)
- Absolute indications for amputation in open tibial fractures- warm ischemia time >6 hrs, tibial nerve avulsion *[handwritten: loss of plantar sensation]*
- Avulsion amputations- cannot replant due to extended area of neurovascular damage
- Lower extremity replantation indication- young patient with both legs cleanly amputated. Contraindications- crush, ischemia >8 hrs, multi-level injury, poor health, old
- 6 inch stump of proximal tibia is needed for prosthetic
- Vascularized bone graft- defects >6cm, infection, prior failure of non-vascularized graft
- BMP- osteoinductive, approved for >12 years. Iliac bone graft- osteoconductive & osteoinductive
- Soleus muscle- broad, posterior calf. Origin- upper 1/3 fibula, medial tibia. Inserts- calcaneus via Achilles tendon. Blood supply- peroneal artery proximal, posterior tibial artery distal. Innervation- tibial nerve. Pedicled muscle flap for coverage of middle 1/3 lower leg defects
- Sartorius muscle- type IV vascularization, 8-10 pedicles off SFA, enters muscle medially
- Gastrocnemius flap- muscle or musculocutaneous flap. Medial & lateral heads can be used independently. Medial head is longer, more inferior. Lateral- possible footdrop *[handwritten: Common peroneal N.]*
- ALT flap- based descending branch of lateral circumflex femoral artery. Traverses vastus lateralis or between rectus femoris & vastus lateralis. Up to 10x25cm
- Fibula flap- good blood supply, harvest with skin paddle, good if smoker. Pre-op evaluation- doppler for flow-limiting lesions, monophasic signals

- Medial plantar flap- plantar calcaneus coverage. Sensation- medial plantar nerve. Blood supply- medal plantar artery
- Medial gastroc flap- blood supply- medial sural artery. Covers upper 1/3 leg & distal knee. Sensate if saphenous nerve harvested
- Medial soleus flap- blood supply- posterior tibial artery. Motor only- posterior tibial nerve. Covers middle 1/3 leg
- Radial forearm flap- blood supply- radial artery. Sensate if medial or lateral antebrachial cutaneous nerves harvested
- Reverse sural artery flap- based on peroneal artery perforators, 5cm proximal to lateral malleolus. Up to 12×15cm, covers ankle & heel wounds. MC complication- partial flap loss. Modifications- <2 cm pedicle, maintaining mesentery between sural nerve & fascia

Dorsum of foot ←

- Dorsalis pedis flap- blood supply- dorsalis pedis artery. Sensate flap if superficial peroneal nerve harvested. Covers anterior ankle, dorsal distal foot
- Propeller flaps- defects of lower leg & foot. Based on peroneal artery perforators for lateral defects & posterior tibial artery perforators for medial defects. Not reliable for large or lateral foot defects
- Peroneal nerve palsy- footdrop, paresthesia. MC cause- supracondylar femoral fracture, knee dislocation, proximal tibial fracture. S/S- no dorsal foot sensation (first webspace), EHL & tibialis anterior weakness. Dx- electrodiagnostic testing within 1 month. If partial, most will recover. If no improvement in 3 months, decompression performed- neurolysis, direct repair or nerve grafting
- Common peroneal nerve compression- 3rd MC nerve compression syndrome (behind carpal & cubital tunnel). Deep peroneal branch- anterior compartment muscle weakness, superficial peroneal branch- superolateral foot paresthesias
- Superficial peroneal nerve- lateral leg compartment, motor to peroneus longus & brevis, sensory to lateral leg. Injury- lateral leg anesthesia & weakness of eversion & plantar flexion of foot. Spares anterior compartment muscles
- Deep peroneal nerve- motor to tibialis anterior, EHL, EDL, EDB, peroneus tertius. Sensory to 1st web space. Injury- weakness of foot dorsiflexion
- Common peroneal nerve injury @ knee- MC etiology- trauma. S/S- footdrop, no dorsiflexion or ankle eversion, 1st webspace numb, weakness of anterior & lateral compartment muscles
- Femoral nerve- innervates anterior thigh muscles (quads, iliacus, sartorius). Injury- weakness of leg extension
- Obturator nerve- innervates medial thigh muscles (adductor brevis, longus, magnus, gracilis, obturator externus). Sensation of medial thigh. Injury- weakness of thigh adduction & ↓ sensation of medial thigh
- Tibial nerve- sciatic nerve branch. Travels with posterior tibial artery. Motor- gastroc, soleus, plantaris, popliteus, flexor digitorum longus, tibialis posterior, flexor hallucis longus. Sensation- plantar foot. Injury- weakness of plantar flexion, numb plantar foot

- Posterior tibial nerve- motor to posterior calf muscles- ankle plantar flexion, toe flexion. Medial & lateral plantar nerve branches- motor innervation of deep plantar muscles of foot, plantar foot sensation
- Sural nerve- purely sensory, diameter 3-4mm, easy harvest, minimal donor deficit of lateral foot & ankle. Up to 30cm long. Location- 1cm posterior to lateral malleolus
- Greater saphenous vein- between medial malleolus & EHL tendon
- Posterior tibial vessels- between medial malleolus & Achilles tendon
- Dorsalis pedis artery- between tibialis anterior & EHL tendons
- Lateral calcaneal artery- terminal branch of peroneal artery
- Lateral circumflex femoral artery- sartorius, rectus femoris , $A LT/\text{vost} \cdots$ (descending branch), tensor fascia lata (ascending branch)
- Superior & inferior gluteal arteries- gluteus maximus
- First dorsal metatarsal artery (FDMA)- variable anatomy- 2/3 artery from dorsalis pedis, 1/3 from deep plantar artery. Proper digital arteries- distal continuations of FDMA
- Biphasic, triphasic arterial waveforms- good. Monophasic- ↑ risk of ischemia. Toe pressures better indicator of ischemia than ankle pressures. If <30mmHg, get pre-op angiogram
- Osteomyelitis- debridement of bone & soft tissue followed by coverage
- Use lower extremity plantaris tendon for multiple or long upper extremity tendon grafts. Present in 80% of limbs. Harvest with vertical incision anterior to medial Achilles tendon (close to tibial nerve)
- Amniotic band syndrome- caused by early amnion rupture & entanglement of fetal parts by strand. Range from simple constrictions to major visceral defects. Extremities- asymmetric digital ring constrictions, distal atrophy, intrauterine amputations, acrosyndactyly, lymphedema, clubfoot. Incidence 1:1200-5000 births. M=F. RF-prematurity, ↓ birth weight, maternal illness, drug exposure, hemorrhage, attempted abortion. No genetic association
- Toe syndactyly- no dysfunction, repair optional
- Zone of polarizing activity- signals limb bud anterior→posterior
- Apical ectodermal ridge- proximal→distal limb growth. Deletion of gene results in shortened limb. SE of maternal retinoids
- Thalidomide- phocomelia, dysmelia, amelia, bone hypoplasticity. Due to vasculogenesis interference
- Congenital talipes equinovarus- aka clubfoot- preoperative tissue expanders can allow primary closure of release sites
- Tarsal tunnel- tibial nerve bifurcates into medial & lateral plantar nerves
- Sensory neuropathy- coordination loss, ↑ mechanical stress, unperceived trauma, Charcot foot, ulcers
- Sympathetic neuropathy- warm, dry, skin breakdown
- Arterial ulcers- male, atherosclerosis, CV disease, DM, HTN, smoking. S/S- claudication, rest pain, non-bleeding, punched-out ulcer. Better with leg dependent, worse with elevation. If ABI <0.45 must revascularize
- Venous stasis ulcer- valve incompetence →chronic venous hypertension, ↑ capillary hydrostatic pressure, leakage of fluid into

extracellular space, ↓ oxygen, cellular necrosis, ulceration. Rx- compression (↓ pressure, ↑ oxygen delivery, ↑ wound healing) +/- unna wrap, HBO, vac

42. Chest Wall / Abdominal Wall

- Post-sternotomy wound classification
  - Type I- 1st week, no bony involvement
  - Type II- 2nd- 4th weeks, frequently has bony involvement
  - Type III- months-years, osteomyelitis, chostochondritis & retained foreign bodies
- Sternal wound infection- debridement, sternal closure, wound closure +/- flaps. Pectoralis flap (thoracoacromial artery), omental flap with STSG, or rectus flap (intercostal artery)
- Thoracic intercostal nerves- nerve grafts up to 12cm with minimal donor site numbness
- Intrinsic chest muscles- external intercostal, internal intercostal, innermost intercostal, and transverse thoracis muscles. External intercostal is most active during inspiration.
- Intercostal nerve exits spinal cord, splits into dorsal & ventral rami
- Component separation- division of external oblique fascia lateral to linea semilunaris (lateral border of rectus sheath). Rectus muscle remains innervated because the internal oblique layer shields the nerve. Rectus muscle turnover flap provides extra coverage but divides intercostal nerves- motor supply to the rectus. Measurements- 10cm epigastrium, 20cm mid-abdomen, 6cm low abdomen
- Loss of domain Rx- component separation & mesh reinforcement
- Pedicled ALT flap- full-thickness abdominal wall reconstruction if component separation not an option
- Myelomeningocele repair- need layer of soft-tissue between dura & skin repairs (paraspinous muscle advancement flaps)
- Posterior thigh flap- posterior femoral cutaneous nerve (S1-S3). Descending branch of the inferior gluteal artery. Coverage- posterior aspect of the thigh, pelvis, vagina
- Superficial epigastric & superficial external pudendal arteries from femoral artery
- Midabdomen- deep epigastric arcade. Lower abdomen- epigastric arcade & external iliac artery
- Inferior epigastric artery runs on posterior rectus sheath
- Intercostal, subcostal, lumbar arteries serve flanks & lateral abdomen
- Deep circumflex iliac artery supplies muscles around ASIS
- VRAM flap- treats APR or vagina defects. Easy to harvest, minimal morbidity, good skin paddle, blood supply, arc of rotation
- Vaginal defects- VRAM, gracilis, pudendal artery fasciocutaneous, deep inferior epigastric artery perforator, interpositional colonic grafts & skin grafting. Return to sexual activity is variable. MC complication- stenosis. Less common- abdominal hernia, rectovaginal fistula, pelvic abscess, small-bowel obstruction

- Pudendal thigh flap (Singapore flap)- thin, sensate, local fasciocutaneous flap used for neovaginal reconstruction. Based on posterior labial arteries. Endovaginal hair growth Rx- pre-op laser
- Congenital absence of vagina- bilateral pudendal fasciocutaneous flaps based on superficial perineal vessels
- Labiaplasty- avoid direct amputation & anterior scar due to pain. Instead use incisions placed inferior, medial, or transverse
- Dorsal nerve of clitoris (from pudendal nerve) is analogous to dorsal nerve of penis. Used for neurorrhaphy with penile reconstruction
- Penile replantation- repair urethra & 3 neurovascular structures- dorsal nerves, veins & artery. Suprapubic catheter for 2-3 weeks
- Gender identity disorder- first step is referral to psychiatrist
- Urachal sinus- red, draining belly button. Rx- surgical excision

43. Skin, Fat & Cartilage Grafts

- Allograft- aka homograft. Nonidentical human. Eventually rejects
- Autograft- from the same patient
- Isograft- genetically identical donor, twin
- Xenograft- cross-species graft. Temporary skin substitutes
- FTSG- contains epidermis & dermis, ↓ contracture. Must defat the graft
- STSG- do not include entire dermis , ↑ long-term contracture. Thickness 8-14/1000inch. +/- meshing (↑ contracture)
- STSG donor site heals spontaneously from epithelial appendages in dermis & wound edges. Starts within 24hrs. Rate directly proportional to # of epithelial appendages & inversely proportional to thickness
- STSG survival- 24hrs by serum imbibition. At 24hrs, vessels invade graft (inosculation). Circulation established by day 4. Graft maturation, collagen turnover in months
- Hematoma- MC skin graft loss. Prevent by meshing, but contraction & poor cosmesis
- Skin grafts directly on tenosynovium limits tendon excursion
- Donor site dressing- promotes rapid re-epithelialization, ↓ pain, requires little care, inexpensive, ↓ infection rate. Options- occlusive dressings (Duoderm), semi-occlusive dressings (OpSite, Tegaderm), semi-open dressings (Xeroform), no dressing. Best is semi-occlusive- fastest healing rates, lowest pain, infection rate, cost. Fluid collections promote moist wound healing
- Dermal fat grafts- harvested like FTSG. Abdomen, gluteal or inframammary folds, subiliac crest, forearm
- Cultured epidermal autografts- patient's keratinocytes expanded in culture in 2-3wks. No elasticity- stiff wounds, blisters, shearing, cost, delay
- Fat graft survival- atraumatic harvesting, placing small aliquots in lattice-like framework, well-vascularized recipient site. Better fat graft survival in supramuscular layer than in subcutaneous & submuscular layers. 30-70% resorption

- Facial fat injection complications- blindness & stroke. Fragments reach ocular & cerebral arteries via carotid arteries. Immediate or delayed presentation. Perform slowly with low force
- Fat necrosis on mammogram- lipid cysts, spiculated masses & round, punctate, diffuse microcalcifications
- Mycobacteria infection after fat grafting- cellulitis & abscess without fever. Dx- PCR. Cultures can be negative
- Autologous cartilage of septum, concha, or rib is ideal donor. ↓ infection, extrusion
- Cartilage grafts with intact perichondrium can curl. Must harvest in subperichondrial plane. Symmetrical graft design ↓ warping. Wait 30 min after carving graft to allow initial warping to occur. Central cuts are less likely to warp than peripheral cuts. Suture will not prevent warping. Low metabolic rate of cartilage, therefore minimal volume loss
- Ear cartilage harvest complications- hematoma, sensory impairment (concha). Cosmesis complications are rare
- Costal cartilage harvest complication- pneumothorax. Dx- intra-op Valsalva maneuver. Rx- evacuate air, no need for chest tube
- Donor for nasal dorsum- costal cartilage. Available, naturally straight. Internal stabilization with K-wires can prevent graft warping
- Exposed silicone nasal prosthesis- replace with cartilage graft
- Osteogenesis- mechanism of cancellous & vascularized bone grafts. Osteoblasts produce new bone @ recipient site
- Osteoconduction- aka creeping substitution. Mechanism of cortical bone grafts. Nonviable scaffold blood vessel ingrowth. Resorption & replacement of graft with new bone
- Osteoinduction- recipient mesenchymal cells stimulated to differentiate into bone-producing cells
- Osseointegration- direct chemical bonding to bony surface
- Endochondral ossification- fracture callus transforms into bone
- Cancellous bone graft- more osteoconductive, osteoinductive, remodeled, revascularized. Bridge bone gaps <5cm
- Cortical bone graft- >2 months to revascularize
- Integra- dermal substitute bilayer of bovine tendon collagen-glycosaminoglycan matrix. Host tissue infiltrates dermal layer, forms neodermis that accepts STSG. Advantages- cosmesis, ↓ contracture, scar, availability, large quantities, elasticity, avoid microsurgical procedure, placement over tendons. Disadvantages- cost, learning curve, multiple stages, infection
- Acellular allogeneic dermis- human cadaveric allograft skin. Type IV & VII collagen & laminin. Ingrowth of host fibroblasts & endothelial cells
- Diabetic foot ulcer biologic dressings- Apligraf, OrCel- bilayered bovine collagen with human keratinocytes & fibroblasts. Releases growth factors & proteins to encourage wound healing
- Santyl- enzymatic degradation of wound bed
- Parry-Romberg syndrome- involves bone, cartilage, fat, skin. Rx- free tissue transfer, fat grafting

cusp de subn

- Craniofacial reconstruction after infection, tumor, trauma- autologous bone grafts are gold standard- good healing, ↓ infection. Drawbacks- unpredictable resorption, donor site morbidity, long operative times, difficult to contour
- Methylmethacrylate- calvarial reconstruction. Drawbacks- infection, fracture, lack of integration, difficulty shaping, heat-induced tissue necrosis
- Hydroxyapatite- capable of osteoconduction & osseointegration. Isothermic, easy to use, maintains volume over time, no xray scatter, ↓ infection
- Pediatric cranium reconstruction- autogenous bone. Calvarial bone preferred (in operative field, good volume retention & strength). Calvarial bone cannot split until 4 years old. Cranial particulate bone grafting- tiny pieces of bone harvested with hand-driven bit which can be done at any age

44. Skin Lesions

- Apocrine glands- axillae, groin, perineum. Secrete viscous, milky fluid, malodorous. If occluded- inflammation, abscess, pain, drainage, foul odor
- Eccrine glands- all skin. Secrete thin, clear, hypotonic fluid (sweat)
- Glomus bodies- fingertips, ears
- Sebaceous glands- secrete sebum, lubricates hair follicles, skin. All skin except palms & soles, many in face & scalp
- Meissner & Vater-Pacini corpuscles- dermal neural mechanoreceptors in glabrous skin
- Palmar & regular skin both have- intraepidermal nerve endings, sweat ducts & glands, irregular border between epidermis & dermis, network of blood vessels, sensory & autonomic nerve fibers in dermis. Palmar skin- deeper papillae & ridges, thicker keratin layer, no pilosebaceous structures
- BCC
  - pearly white with telangiectasias, or pimple-like sore that bleeds, heals & recurs
  - <2cm only needs 3mm margin for 95% cure
  - medical Rx- 5-FU, cryotherapy, XRT
  - morpheaform BCC- "finger-like" extensions seen histologically, therefore ↑ recurrence rate with simple excision. Rx- Mohs
  - Excision of BCC with undermining- code for malignant excision & complex closure. Excision of BCC with local flap closure- code for adjacent tissue transfer only, not malignant excision
- Nevoid basal cell carcinoma (Gorlin) syndrome- AD. Presents at birth or childhood. S/S- tan papules on face, neck, trunk, palm & plantar foot pits, molar area edema & pain (odontogenic keratocysts),

colobomas, hypertelorism, fibrosarcomas. Dx- biopsy. Rx- excision, 5-FU, imiquimod, frequent examinations

- Bazex syndrome- AD. Multiple BCCs of face, follicular atrophoderma of extremities, hypohidrosis, hypotrichosis
- Pyogenic granuloma- childhood, rapidly growing, red lesion, <1cm, bleeds. Rx- excision
- Keloid Rx- excision +/- XRT. SE- hypo/hyperpigmentation, telangiectasias
- Purpura fulminans- autoimmune septic shock, hemorrhagic bullae, desquamation, fatal. Usually Neisseria meningitides. Rx- recognize fast, antibiotics, supportive care, fasciotomy improves limb salvage. If develop DIC, Rx is activated protein C. No surgery until demarcated
- Merkel cell carcinoma- smooth, painless, indurated, solitary nodule, 2-4mm in size. MC >65 years old, sun-exposed areas. Half are head & neck. Very aggressive, metastases & local recurrence common. 5-year survival 30-60%. Rx- same as melanoma margins (except tumor width determines margins, not depth), SLNBx, XRT
- Desmoid tumors- benign tumors of abdominal wall. Locally invasive, high recurrence rate. Rx- WLE with 1cm margin
- Keratoacanthoma- low-grade malignancy, resembles SCC. Grows fast then regresses over several months. Can progress to SCC with metastasis
- Cutaneous horn- hyperkeratosis over a skin lesion (seborrheic or actinic keratosis)
- Hidradenitis suppurativa- subcutaneous nodules, puberty, F>M, rupture or coalesce, deep, painful abscesses, sinus tracts. Rx- hygiene, antibiotics (clindamycin, tetracycline). Severe Rx- wide excision of all affected tissue
- Actinic keratosis- common, premalignant lesion, sun damage, fair-skinned patients, flat or slightly raised, red, scaly. 25% progress to SCC, Bowen disease, cutaneous horns, keratoacanthomas. Rx- sunscreen, 5FU cream, imiquimod cream (Aldara), cryotherapy, photodynamic therapy with 5-aminolevulinic acid (Levulan)
- Seborrheic keratosis- middle-aged & older patients, sharp borders, waxy, friable, look stuck-on, tan to black. Rx- shave excision, electrodesiccation, freezing, excision. No malignant degeneration
- Dermatofibroma- benign, anterior leg, asymptomatic, firm, 3-10mm, any color. Dx- Fitzpatrick sign- dimpling of lesion with lateral compression. Suspect lupus if >15 lesions. Rx- cosmetic or unsure of diagnosis- excisional biopsy
- Calcinosis cutis- calcification of soft tissues & skin. Painful, ulcerate, drainage, infection. MC- extremity joints, bony prominences. Deposits in dermis. Rx- surgical excision. Distinct from calciphylaxis
- Calciphylaxis- poorly understood, highly morbid, vascular calcification, skin necrosis in ESRD patients. Debridement makes worse
- Xeroderma pigmentosum- AR. Defective DNA repair. ↑ cancer risk. Multiple skin malignancies can start in youth. Severe sunburn that lasts weeks in toddler, many early freckles, irregular dark spots, thin skin, dryness, solar keratoses, skin cancers, sensitive eyes to light,

CREST
syndrome ←
↑
Scleroderma

blistering or freckling with small amount of sun exposure, premature aging, crusting, raw skin. Rx- minimize sun exposure, isotretinoin, cryotherapy, 5-FU, multiple excisions

- Erythroplasia of Queyrat- Bowen disease of glans penis, uncircumcised men, SCC in situ
- Rhinophyma- red/purple nose with telangiectasias, pits, fissures, scarring, enlarged nasal tip, hypertrophic nasal skin, secondary nasal airway obstruction
- Facial dermatitis- MC perioral, young women. Erythematous micropapules form inflammatory plaques
- Dermoid cyst- mass with distinct margins, no intracranial extension, lateral upper orbit. Rx- excision. If <u>proptosis or lesion ↓ in size with palpation</u>, cyst may extend orbital wall-order CT (midline cysts MC intracranial involvement)
- Chondrodermatitis nodularis helicis- chronic, inflammatory, painful, nodular lesion of helix or antihelix. Interferes with sleep. Path- focal cartilage degeneration, perichondritis. Etiology unknown. Rx- steroid injections, excision
- Tricholemmoma- benign scalp tumor, looks like epidermal inclusion cyst. Rx- excision
- Nevus of Ota- blue-gray lesion of face in trigeminal nerve distribution. MC in female blacks. Dx- biopsy. Rx- Q-switched ruby laser, eye examination. 4% melanoma risk
- Nevus of Ito- similar to nevus of Ota but in lateral brachial cutaneous & supraclavicular nerves distribution
- Nevus sebaceus of Jadassohn- yellow-orange plaque of face or scalp. BCC potential
- Lymphangioma circumscriptum- clusters of clear-white vesicular lesions, obliterate with gentle pressure then refill with lymph. MC-upper arm, axilla, pectoral, scapula areas. Rx- excision skin & lymphatics
- Blue rubber bleb nevi- raised blue rubbery lesion, compressible. Malformed vascular channels of skin & bowel. If blood removed→wrinkled sac→refills with blood. Rx- excision if painful
- Dermatosis papulosa nigra- seborrheic keratosis variant of blacks & Asians. Begin in adolescence, cheek area. Rx- shave excision, curettage, cryotherapy
- Melasma- hyperpigmentation of face, neck from pregnancy or estrogen
- Epidermal inclusion cyst- aka sebaceous cyst. Proliferation of epidermal cells within the dermis. Anywhere on body, benign, cyst wall is stratified squamous epithelium, slow-growing, can become infected. Rx- excision of entire cyst or will recur
- Angiosarcoma- rare, highly aggressive tumor. MC- face & scalp in old white men. Can look like bruise or cellulitis, multifocal, local recurrence common. Rx- WLE + XRT. Preoperative punch biopsies help establish margins
- Trichoepitheliomas- multiple, benign, yellow-pink papules of cheeks, eyelids, nasolabial area. F>M. Rx- none. Desmoplastic trichoepithelioma- biopsy to rule out cancer

- Eccrine poroma- MC palm or sole, >40 years old, <2cm, rare malignant transformation. Rx- excision
- Verrucous nevus- verrucous papules coalesce into plaques. Can be linear along skin tension lines. Path- hyperkeratosis, acanthosis, papillomatosis. Rx- excision if amenable, laser cryotherapy, dermabrasion
- Cylindroma- solitary or multiple benign lesions. MC- face. Adulthood. Rx- excision, electrosurgery
- Nevus sebaceous- MC scalp, forehead, retroauricular. Single, waxy, yellow, asymptomatic, epithelial & nonepithelial skin components. 2/3 seen at birth. M=F. Rx- excision before puberty due to possible progression to BCC (5%)
- Dermatofibrosarcoma protuberans- rare. MC cutaneous sarcoma. Malignant tumor of dermis, slow-growing, MC- trunk, irregular shape, infiltrating growth pattern. Rx- excision with 2cm margins (local recurrence common), Mohs in sensitive areas +/- XRT, Gleevec if unresectable or metastatic. SLNBx not indicated
- Pyoderma gangrenosum- small, painful, red-purple plaque of lower extremity after minor trauma which progresses to ulcer. Probably immune-related (associated with ulcerative colitis, Crohn's, rheumatoid arthritis). Rx- steroids, immunosuppression, surgery is last resort & may exacerbate
- Marjolin ulcer- SCC of long-standing wound or burn scar. Rx- resection
- Leishmaniasis- parasitic disease spread by sand fly. Skin ulcer at bite. Dx- history of insect bite, travel to Central & South America, West Asia, Middle East), seeing organisms under the microscope
- Scleroderma- autoimmune fibrosis of the skin. Limited- Raynaud's, distal tip ulceration, thin, tight skin over joints. Systemic- GI, pulmonary, renal, cardiac fibrosis
- Necrotizing fasciitis- rapidly spreading soft-tissue infection, travels along fascial planes, mono- or polymicrobial, MC- Group A Strep, Staph aureus, B. frag, Clostridium. Rx- IV antibiotics, debridement
- Stewart-Treves syndrome- lymphangiosarcoma in postmastectomy patients. Chronic wound looks like radionecrosis. Dx- incisional biopsy. 5-year survival <1%. Rx- surgery & isolated limb perfusion with tumor necrosis factor & melphalan
- Cutis laxa- hypoelastic skin that doesn't spring back. Defect of elastin fibers. Congenital or acquired. ↑ hernia risk. Normal scar & healing. May need to repeat rhytidectomy & blepharoplasty
- Ehlers-Danlos syndrome- aka cutis hyperelastica. S/S- skin hyperextensibility, joint laxity, tissue friability, skin springs back, ventral hernias, wide, thin scars. MC inherited collagen disorder. Wound or anastomosis dehiscence @ 1-2 wks
- Osler-Weber-Rendu syndrome- malformed vessels of skin, mucous membranes, viscera after puberty & ↑ age. Bleeding lesions- epistaxis, hematemesis, hematuria, melena
- Neurofibromatosis- aka- von Recklinghausen's. AD. Lesion- schwann cells, fibroblasts, mast cells. Iris hamartomas (Lisch nodules), axillary freckling, acoustic neuromas, meningiomas, mental retardation,

Sarcoma ↓ hematogenous (handwritten margin note, next to Dermatofibrosarcoma)

CREST (handwritten margin note, next to Scleroderma)

pheochromocytomas. 3-15% malignant. Rx- excise if rapidly growing or painful
- Organ transplant SE- diabetes, obesity, gout, osteoporosis, atherosclerosis, malignant skin tumors, lymphoproliferative disorders, fungal & bacterial infections
- Mohs indications-
    o recurrent or incompletely excised BCC, SCC
    o BCC, SCC with indistinct borders in cosmetic or functional high-risk areas
    o aggressive clinical behavior or histologic subtype
    o undifferentiated or poorly differentiated SCC
    o area of previous XRT
    o lesions of immunosuppressed patients
    o basal cell nevus syndrome patients Gorlin syndrome
- Imiquimod (Aldara)- immune enhancer, induces apoptosis of tumor cells. Rx for- AK, BCC, SCC, viral warts
- Topical 5-FU- chemo that inhibits DNA synthesis
- Retinoids- prevents skin cancer by regulating cell differentiation
- Topical diclofenac- anti-inflammatory. Rx for AK
- Interferons- modifies gene transcription. Use with retinoids for advanced SCC

45. Hemangiomas

- Hemangiomas- vascular tumors with ↑ cellular proliferation, rapid growth, slow regression. MC- tumor in infancy, girls, premature infants. Extracutaneous- parotid glands, liver. Can be proceded with telangiectasia or bruise-like patch (herald patch)
- Intramuscular hemangioma- rapidly growing vascular lesion not present at birth, diagnostic challenges, no cutaneous changes. Rx- propranolol, corticosteroids
- Hemangioma Rx- Nonulcerating, nonobstructive- observe. Ulcerating, obstructing- systemic or intralesional corticosteroid, oral prednisone, interferon, pulsed-dye laser or resection. Surgery only for lesions that don't respond to medical management or that compromise function (pain or nerve compression)
- Congenital hemangioma- fully grown at birth. 2 types- rapidly involuting congenital hemangioma (RICH) & noninvoluting congenital hemangioma (NICH). RICH- gone in 12 months, no Rx. NICH- steady size for life, Rx rarely needed
- Lip hemangioma- early surgery for infantile hemangiomas & vascular malformations. Linear closure along vertical resting tension lines
- Periocular hemangioma- can cause eyelid ptosis, visual field obstruction, strabismus, anisometropia, astigmatism, amblyopia, blindness. Rx- propranolol first. Surgical indications- easy to resect, astigmatism, visual obstruction, medical treatment failure. Best visual outcome if resected before 3 months old
- Parotid gland hemangioma Rx- systemic corticosteroid

- Vascular malformation- present at birth, grow slowly. M=F. Dx- US, CT, MRI. Rx- sclerotherapy or resection
- Kaposiform hemangioendothelioma- malignant vascular tumor present at birth, stable size, red-purple color, tense, shiny, large, superficial, on trunk or extremities, can have Kasabach-Merritt thrombocytopenia, bruising, bleeding. Rx- vincristine +/- surgery (no more interferon alfa-2a due to spastic diplegia)
- Pseudoaneurysm- due to acute external or internal injury that disrupts the endothelium & bleeds
- True aneurysm- endothelial-lined widening of artery with all 3 layers of vessel intact. Fusiform, dilated. Due to repetitive or blunt trauma, Kawasaki disease, arteriosclerosis, hemophilia
- Branham sign- slowing pulse upon compression proximal to arteriovenous malformation
- Traumatic arteriovenous fistula- MRA for pre-op planning
- Maffucci syndrome- venous malformations & multiple enchondromas, possible malignant chondrosarcomas & intracranial tumors (20%)
- Sturge-Weber syndrome- facial capillary malformations (port-wine stain) in 1st & 2nd trigeminal nerve distribution. MRI- vascular anomalies of leptomeninges & choroid plexus. Can also have seizure disorders
- Parkes-Weber syndrome- variant of Klippel-Trenaunay syndrome. Port-wine stains of lower extremity, lymphatic/venous malformations, hypertrophy, arteriovenous fistulae
- Osler-Weber-Rendu syndrome- aka hereditary hemorrhagic telangiectasia syndrome. AD. Face, tongue, lips, nasal & oral mucosa, conjunctiva, hands/nails. Occur later in life
- Cobb syndrome- capillary malformation of scalp overlying encephalocele or dysraphism of cervical or lumbosacral spine
- Klippel-Tranaunay syndrome- capillary-lymphatic-venous malformation. Unilateral extremity +/- thorax hypertrophy. Dark red staining with vesicles. Embryonal lateral vein of Servelle in lower extremity. Risk of DVT, PE
- Nevus flammeus neonatorum- resolved by 1 year old. Upper face, posterior neck
- Venous malformation Rx- sclerotherapy, excision (very morbid, scar)
- Symptomatic AVM Rx- radical excision
- Lymphatic malformation- MC neck & axilla. Rx- sclerotherapy, resection only if symptomatic after sclerotherapy
- Percutaneous sclerotherapy- Rx low-flow arteriovenous & lymphatic malformations
- Pulsed-dye laser- Rx thin, vascular lesions. Multiple treatments, painful, residual scarring
- Intralesional bleomycin- multiple treatments with anesthesia
- Propranolol- 1 mg/kg TID, start IV with monitoring, then transition to PO. Dramatic responses in 1 day, resolution in few weeks. Contraindications- bronchospasm, cardiac abnormalities, cerebrovascular abnormalities. MC SE- lethargy, hypoglycemia, ↓ BP, ↓ pulse. Most effective for early lesions in proliferative growth phase

- Oral prednisolone complications- short-term cushingoid facies (MC), personality changes, gastric irritation, fungal infections, hyperglycemia, 2 years for growth to catch up after long treatment (9-12 months)

46. Melanoma

- Melanocytic hyperplasia without atypia is benign. Rx- observe
- Lentigo maligna- melanoma in situ, sun-exposed elderly, slow-growing. Rx- excise with 1cm margins. Do not use imiquimod or lasers due to recurrence risk
- Intermediate-thickness melanomas- 25% risk of regional disease. Before SLNBx, elective lymphadenectomy was done, with most being negative
- Congenital nevomelanocytic lesion- 5-12% risk of malignancy, half of melanomas occur within nevi, half within CNS or normal skin
- Giant nevi- half occur by age 3 & most by puberty. >20 cm in adults, or 9cm on head, 6cm on body of child). ↑ risk of melanoma. Rx- serial excision
- Neurocutaneous melanosis- GCM, hydrocephalus, seizures, focal deficits, partial paresis. Occurs before age 2. Dx- MRI. Rx- surgery after age 2
- Amelanotic melanoma- uncommon, nonpigmented, appear pink or tan, mimics BCC & SCC
- Nail bed lesion- shave biopsy. Core biopsy causes nail bed abnormality
- Nail atypia or melanoma in situ Rx- excision with clear margins. Close with full- or split-thickness nail bed graft
- Acral lentiginous melanoma- under nail, palm of hand, sole of foot. Prognosis worse, due to delay in diagnosis
- Subungual hand melanoma- 5-year survival only 30%. Rx- amputation through joint proximal to lesion. Close with volar flaps
- Breslow tumor thickness is most important predictor of local recurrence, metastases, overall survival
- Excisional margins
    - 0.5-1cm for melanoma in situ/lentigo maligna, invasive lesions <1mm
    - 1-2cm for 1-2mm
    - 2 cm for >2 mm, aggressive pathology (ulceration, lymphovascular invasion, tumor regression, ↑ mitotic index
- SLNBx- melanoma with aggressive pathology, males with truncal melanoma <0.76mm thick, all patients with melanomas >.76mm, SCC >2cm, merkel cell carcinoma, marjolin ulcer. Not for melanoma in situ, BCC, or palpable adenopathy

- Wound healing phases- inflammation→collagen synthesis→angiogenesis→ epithelialization→remodeling
- Cell arrival order in acute wound- platelets→neutrophils→macrophages→ lymphocytes→fibroblasts
- Neutrophils- first leukocytes to appear, cause acute inflammation, peaks @ 24hrs, then macrophages & lymphocytes appear
- Fibroblastic phase- 3-5 days post-injury. Fibroblasts lay new collagen. Type III collagen predominates early then type I
- Epithelial cell migration- initiated by loss of contact inhibition, occurs from wound periphery. Thin layer over wound in 2-3 days. Surgical incision covered 1 day, then can get wet
- Myofibroblasts- wound contraction
- Procollagen cleaved to form collagen→crosslinks to form fibril→weaves to become fiber
- Proline & lysine hydroxylate to form procollagen. Many cofactors needed. Altered in diseases like Ehlers-Danlos
- Peak post-injury tensile strength of skin- 60 days. 80% of original strength
- Inhibit wound repair- antilymphocyte therapy- lymphocyte immune globulin (Atgam), thymoglobulin, basiliximab, antimetabolites-azathioprine, mycophenolate mofetil, calcineurin inhibitors-cyclosporine, FK-506, glucocorticosteroids
- Keloid scars extend beyond original scar. ↑ fibroblast proliferation rates. ↓ blood vessels. No myofibroblasts. Rx- XRT ↓ recurrence rates to 12-27%. SE- pigmentary changes
- Hypertrophic scar Rx- observe
- Pressure garments for fibroproliferative scars- local tissue hypoxia, ↓ fibroblast proliferation & collagen synthesis
- Split cranial bone graft healing is by osteoconduction. Graft is mostly cortical- scaffold for blood vessels & osteoprogenitor cells. Creeping substitution replacement of graft with new bone
- Spontaneous dural ossification- heals full-thickness cranial defects in infants
- Osteogenesis- mechanism of bone graft healing in cancellous or vascularized bone grafts. Revascularize rapidly & osteoblasts make new bone
- Osteoinduction- stimulation of recipient site mesenchymal cells to differentiate into bone-producing cells. Ex- demineralized bone, bone morphogenetic protein
- Integra- bovine collagen bilaminate neodermal replacement. Glycosaminoglycan matrix with silicone outer layer. Used in burn reconstruction, exposed bone without periosteum, exposed cartilage without perichondrium, exposed tendon without paratenon. Provides scaffold for neovascularization. At 3-4 wks the silicone outer later is removed & STSG
- Biobrane- temporary bilaminar skin substitute with inner nylon & collagen, outer silicone film. Prevents evaporative loss, wound

- desiccation, ↓ pain, provides barrier to bacteria. Remove before grafting or after epithelialization
- Acticoat- silver dressing activated with water. Releases silver 3-7 days
- Dermagraft- neonatal foreskin dermal substitute. Treats diabetic foot ulcers, combined with STSG
- TransCyte- temporary wound dressing. Biobrane + neonatal fibroblasts. Remove before skin grafting or after epithelialization. ↓ pain & time to epithelialization
- Apligraf- permanent replacement made of type I bovine collagen, cultured neonatal human fibroblasts & keratinocytes. Treats venous & diabetic foot ulcers. Can take multiple applications
- Large open wound fails to show healing progress- nutritional evaluation & supplements
- Vitamin C- assists in collagen cross-linking via hydroxylation of proline & lysine. Scurvy- bleeding, loss of dentition, lack of osteoid formation
- Folate & vitamin B6 (pyridoxine)- DNA synthesis & cellular proliferation
- Vitamin A- epithelialization & fibroblast proliferation. Treats glucocorticoid impaired wounds. Rx- 15,000 IU daily x 7 days
- Vitamin E- antioxidant & immune modulator
- Zinc- cofactor for metalloenzymes, proteins & nucleic acid synthesis
- Adriamycin extravasation- severe tissue necrosis. Rx- observe for debridement need
- Radiation effects- free radical production that damages DNA. Acute- erythema, edema, vasodilation, lymphatic obliteration, capillary thrombosis, impaired tissue oxygenation. Chronic- nonhealing ulcers
- Anemia with good circulation doesn't impair wound healing
- Flap closure for full-thickness wound with exposed bone. Need to rid infection & optimize nutrition. Wound vac while waiting
- Wound vac- promotes wound healing by removing excess interstitial fluid, shrinks wound, enhances granulation tissue formation
- HBO therapy- Rx- osteomyelitis, necrotizing infections, ischemia-reperfusion injury, diabetic lower extremity wounds. Do not use for extravasation injury, pressure sores, pyoderma gangrenosum, burns. ↑ antimicrobial activity by ↑ neutrophils, ↑ hyperoxygenation of tissue 10-15x, stimulate angiogenesis, ↓ ischemia-reperfusion injury
- Chronic wounds- ↑ metalloproteinases causes extracellular matrix degradation. ↑ proinflammatory cytokines & ↓ matrix deposition delays epithelization & healing. ↓ oxygen tension in central part of chronic wounds
- Silver ions kill bacteria. No known resistant organisms, but nontoxic to human cells
- Alginates- absorb 20x their weight. Treats exudative wounds
- Silicone gel sheeting- ↑ hydration from occlusion. Wear 12hrs/day x 3 months
- Pressure >40 mmHg for wound healing. Dx- pulsatile plethysmography, transcutaneous oxygen >30 torr. If insufficient-

angiography, revascularization. Do not flap a patient with arterial insufficiency
- 1% povidone-iodine- bactericidal activity without fibroblast toxicity
- Hand & face transplant- monitor skin for acute rejection
- Vascular endothelial-growth factor- ↑ during ischemia. Ex-tissue expansion
- Silicone injection SE- migration, induration, pigment changes, painful subcutaneous nodules, infection, ulceration. Rx- resection & reconstruction. Histology- granulomas
- Histology of capsule around prostheses- acellularity & organized layers of collagen

48. Tissue Expansion

- ↑ cell division via stretch-induced growth factors, cytoskeleton, protein kinases
- ↑ protein synthesis, keratinocytes, new skin production
- MC failure site- scalp. High complication rates in lower leg
- Can cover up to 50% scalp loss. Place in subgaleal plane
- Rectangular & crescent devices expand more than circular devices
- Expand until flap is 20% larger than defect
- Disadvantages- ↑ time, multiple operations, high complication rate, infection, device extrusion, hematoma, flap necrosis, skull erosion, alopecia, poor scarring
- After expansion- thickens epidermis through hyperkeratosis, ↑ collagen & surface area, ↓ tensile strength & elasticity, thinning of dermis, muscle & fat

vascular delay

49. Pressure Sore

- Pressure sore stages:
    o Stage I- intact skin, erythema, warmth, induration, reversible, improves with pressure reduction
    o Stage II- abrasion, blister, superficial ulcer, reversible
    o Stage III- full-thickness skin loss through subcutaneous tissue, not into fascia
    o Stage IV- muscle, bone, tendon, or joint. Osteomyelitis & undermining often present
- Do not treat ulcers if patient is still smoking, non-compliant, malnourished
- Pressure sore caused by prolonged pressure > end capillary pressure (32 mmHg)
- Ischial pressure wound- posterior thigh flap- semimembranosus, semitendinosus & biceps femoris muscles. Reliable, re-advanceable, made in V-Y

- Thoracolumbar or lumbar wound- local flaps unless XRT, extensive trauma, large area- then free tissue transfer indicated. Lat dorsi better than omentum
- Sacral wound- Rotational or advanced gluteal muscle flap. Gluteal fasciocutaneous flap conserves muscle, allows ambulation, less sensitive to ischemia, more resistant to pressure, high mechanical resistance. Lumbosacral flap for stage III, IV ulcers
- Trochanteric wound- TFL muscle-only or with skin. Also consider vastus lateralis flap
- TFL not good for ischial ulcers- distal aspect of flap is too thin to give adequate padding
- Ischial pressure sore in young, ambulatory patient- gluteal fasciocutaneous flap spares muscle
- Posterior thigh fasciocutaneous rotation flap- ambulatory patient, durable, no functional deformity, but not much bulk for large ulcers
- Postoperative regimen- bed rest, pressure-relieving mattress, no sitting for 3 weeks
- Fibrotic pressure sore- impaired wound healing, wound vacs not helpful
- Girdlestone procedure- resection of proximal femur in trochanteric ulcers
- Design flaps that allow future re-advance
- Osteomyelitis Dx- bone biopsy
- Infection- >10 organisms/gram of tissue. Swab cultures are unreliable. Most common complication in pressure sores treated with vac
- Colostomy- reduce soilage in perineal wounds

50. Lymphedema

- Etiology- poor clearance of interstitial fluid. Bilateral lower extremity edema- systemic disease, unilateral edema- venous insufficiency or lymphedema
- MC cause worldwide- filariasis. Wuchereria bancrofti. Travel to Africa
- PE- peau d'orange, Stemmer sign- cannot stent toe skin, blunted digits
- Lymphedema praecox- noncongenital lymphedema that occurs before puberty
- Lymphedema tarda- midlife
- Primary lymphedema- congenital, praecox, or tarda based on age
- Secondary lymphedema- lymphatic obstruction (cancer, infection, XRT) or lymphatic interruption (groin surgery, lymph node excision)
- Massive localized lymphedema- aka lymphedema of obesity. Benign soft tissue overgrowth. Normal lymphatics that have acquired dysfunction. Rx- excision & vac
- Myxedema- thyroid disease. S/S- dry skin, thin hair, ↓ sweat

- Panniculus morbidus- severe abdominal lipodystrophy. Cannot lose weight because cannot exercise, poor hygiene, bad odor, intertrigo, cellulitis, ulceration. Rx- panniculectomy
- Lymphatic malformation- most diagnosed before 2 years. Head & neck, soft, variable size, thin skin, atrophic, or bluish. SE- respiratory compromise
- Milroy's disease- rare, X-linked or AD, primary lymphedema, diagnosed at birth. Unilateral pitting, eye manifestations
- If lymphatic malformation suddenly ↑ in size and tender- infection. Rx- antibiotic
- Rx- hygiene, weight loss, avoid trauma, no tight clothing, elevate extremity, compression garment. Surgery only if fails med management. Improve lymphatic flow & debulk tissue (staged skin & subcutaneous excision)

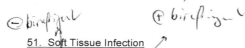

51. Soft Tissue Infection

- Gout & pseudogout- S/S- joint swelling, erythema, pain, fever. Dx- joint aspirate has crystals. Rx- antibiotics, elevation, splinting if indicated
- MC hand infection organism- staph aureus. MC strain- MRSA
- Horseshoe abscess- infection of thumb or small finger travels through wrist into the opposite flexor tendon sheath via Parona space. Rx- explore with extended carpal tunnel release
- Suppurative flexor tenosynovitis- pain over tendon sheath, flexed digit, pain on passive extension, symmetrical finger swelling. MC- staph aureus, eikenella corrodens. Immunocompromised patients- listeria
- Paronychia- infection of space between nail plate & eponychial fold. Causes- nail biting, aggressive manicuring. MC- staph aureus & strep. MC chronic- candida
- Web-space abscess- aka collar-button abscess. S/S- pain with flexion, adduction. Rx- I&D dorsal & volar webspace
- Herpetic whitlow- pain, erythema of fingertip. Dx- Tzanck smear (multinucleated giant cells). Rx- acyclovir
- Tuberculosis tenosynovitis- mycobacterium marinum. Path- nonspecific tenosynovitis, granulomas. Rx- surgery. Rice bodies- on synovial surface which break off inflammatory mass
- Septic joint- analyze synovial fluid
- Disseminated gonococcal infection- MC infectious arthritis in adults. Gram- diplococci. Rx- IV 3rd generation cephalosporin
- Human bite- S aureus, E corrodens, H influenzae, anaerobes. Rx- amoxicillin-clavulanate
- Animal bites- pasteurella
- Horse bite- actinobacillis lignieresii
- Cat bite- polymicrobial, anaerobic organisms, pasteurella multocida. Rx- amoxicillin + clavulanate or penicillin + cephalexin, bactrim + clindamycin or metronidazole, or fluoroquinolone + clindamycin or

metronidazole; debridement, leave open, if possible rabies irrigate with povidone-iodine after wound cultures
- Snake bite- tetanus, observe for envenomation. Rattlesnakes are the most potent & common. Antivenin Rx- worsening local injury, coagulopathy, systemic effects (hypotension, mental status changes). Do not debride or use tourniquets. Fasciotomy if compartment syndrome develops, which is rare
- Leech infections- 2-20%. Cellulitis, necrosis, abscess, or septicemia. MC- aeromonas hydrophila- gram neg anaerobe. Rx- cipro. Prevent-prophylactic antibiotics
- Liposuction is MC surgery associated with necrotizing fasciitis
- Orbital cellulitis- local extension of infection (sinuses, dental or facial abscess). Intraorbital abscess- immediate surgery because risk of blindness. Preseptal cellulitis- superficial to orbital septum. Rx- oral antibiotics. Dx- CT, MRI
- Necrotizing fasciitis- Type I- MC, mixed aerobic & anaerobic infections. Type II- monomicrobic (group A strep, strep pyogenes)
- Cervical necrotizing fasciitis- MC due to pharyngeal or tonsillar infections, dental abscesses. Dx-CT. Rx- broad-spectrum antibiotics, debridement
- Mucormycosis- life-threatening fungal infection. Non-purulent, necrotizing, associated with diabetes. Rx- emergent debridement, culture
- Fournier disease- diabetes, alcoholism, smoker, leukemia, AIDS. Due to urogenital disease, trauma, manipulation. Rx- hydration, broad-spectrum antibiotics, debridement. Orchiectomy is rare- testicles have own blood supply
- Sweet syndrome- acute febrile neutrophilic dermatosis. Non-cellulitic, occurs at sites of minor trauma. Doesn't respond to antibiotics. Rx-steroids
- Sporothrix schenckii- plants, soil. Papule at entry site & lesions up lymphatic chain
- Vibrio vulnificus- gram-negative, coastal US waters handling raw seafood or marine wildlife. S/S- rapid cellulitis, edema, hemorrhagic bullae
- Mastoiditis- mastoid air cell infection due to untreated otitis media. Can spread to brain
- Parotitis- parotid gland infection due to obstructed parotid duct
- Tetanus immune globulin & tetanus toxoid booster - tetanus-prone wound in patient without primary immunization series. If patient has been immunized previously, give booster if last dose >5 years

52. Burns

- Burn center referral- >10% TBSA, involve face, hands, feet, genitalia, perineum, or major joints in young or old patients, all 3rd degree burns, inhalation injury, electrical burns, chemical burns

- Parkland formula for burns > 20% TBSA. 4 mL LR per kg per % TBSA given over 24 hours. 1/2 given in first 8 hours, 1/2 over next 16 hours
- Hourly urine output guides fluid mgmt. Titrate rate to 0.5 mL/kg/hr in adults & 1 mg/kg/hr in children
- 24 hours post-burn add albumin to IVF, since capillary leak is resolved
- ↑ glucose in first 24 hours following burn
- Humoral & cellular-mediated immunity are impaired by thermal injury. ↓ complement immunoglobulins, B-lymphocyte, NKC, T-helper lymphocyte function; ↑ integrins, TNF-a, IL-1, IL-8, T-suppressor lymphocytes
- Zone of coagulation- exposed to the highest temp, irreversible, uniform necrosis of cells. Zone of stasis- surrounds the zone of coagulation, develops ischemia, leading to cell death, injury potentially reversible. Zone of hyperemia- vasodilation, ↑ blood flow, injury is completely reversible. Resuscitate with IVF to prevent converting to another zone
- Diagnose inhalation injury with fiberoptic bronchoscopy
- Burn area splinting- neck in extension, shoulder abducted to 90°, elbow extended to 180°, wrist neutral, hands in intrinsic plus
- Oral commissure burns splinted for 6 months. May bleed from labial artery
- Frostbite
    - freezing of tissues with change in osmotic gradient of cells, causing electrolyte issues. Thromboxanes, prostaglandins, histamine & bradykinin released leads to edema, endothelial injury & tissue damage
    - Rx- rapid rewarming with 104-108°F water for 15-30min, analgesia, elevation, tetanus prophylaxis, debridement of clear blisters, no debridement of hemorrhagic blisters, aloe vera, +/- anticoagulation, thrombolytics, antiprostaglandins (aloe, ibuprofen), HBO, sympathetic blockade
    - treat cellulitis with penicillin
    - tPA- reverses microvascular thrombosis, ↓ amputation rate if given within 24 hours. Follow with systemic heparin
    - Thromboxane A2- tissue damage in frostbite injuries. Ibuprofen blocks the cyclooxygenase cascade that produces thromboxane A2
    - Technetium-99m bone scanning detects level of amputation due to frostbite
- Toxic epidermal necrolysis syndrome- aka TENS, Stevens-Johnson syndrome- exfoliating rash 1-3 weeks after starting medication. Skin sloughs at the dermal-epidermal junction. Mortality- 30%. Rx- transfer to burn center. No topical treatment
- High-voltage injury may develop compartment syndrome. Rx- immediate decompression, including carpal tunnel & pronator quadrates
- MRI used to evaluate muscle damage in electrical injury

- Silvadene- painless. MC SE- transient neutropenia & thrombocytopenia
- Silver nitrate- painless, poor tissue penetration, used in TEN. MC SE- ↓ electrolytes, brown staining of skin, methemoglobinemia
- Sulfamylon- painful, good penetration. MC SE- metabolic acidosis
- Cultured epidermal autografts- used for large wounds with limited donor sites. After taking skin biopsy, tissue is processed by a laboratory. In 3 weeks keratinocytes expand 10,000-fold
- Apligraf- permanent, biosynthetic, bilayered, foreskin-derived neonatal human keratinocytes & fibroblasts cultured on bovine-type collagen. Treat weekly x 5
- AlloDerm- human cryopreserved, acellular, cadaveric, de-epidermalized dermis that repopulates with host fibroblasts & endothelial cells
- Biobrane- type I porcine collagen peptides on silicone film & nylon fabric
- Integra- temporary bilaminate made of silicone & cross-linked bovine tendon collagen & shark-derived glycosaminoglycans. Use to cover tendons
- Surgisis- porcine small intestine made into 3-D matrix of collagen & proteins
- Acticoat- thin layer of silver ion provides antimicrobial activity, ↓ dressing changes, pain & cost
- MC burn wound infection bacteria- MRSA, pseudomonas, klebsiella. Rx- vanc & zosyn
- Z-plasty lengthens a scar, breaks up straight line, shifts soft-tissue contour
- Free-tissue transfer in burn patients done 4-6 weeks after injury. In non-burn pts, free flap within 1 week of injury
- Reverse radial forearm flap used to resurface dorsal hand & fingers
- Ear burns Rx- sulfamylon, monitor for chondritis, auto-amputation
- Tissue expansion- reconstruction of up to 50% scalp defect
- Erythroblasts only present in fetus & newborn. Presence is predictive of fatal outcome
- Hydrofluoric acid burn Rx- calcium gluconate injection
- Phenol burn Rx- mineral oil, polyethylene glycol or vegetable oil
- Alkaline solution results in liquefaction necrosis. Ex- anhydrous ammonia
- SIRS- burn patient with 2 criteria:
  1. Body temperature <36°C or >38.5°C
  2. Heart rate >90
  3. Respirations >20
  4. WBC <4000 or >12,000
- Burn scar hypertrophy Rx- compression garments- ↓ blood flow to active scars, ↓ collagen production
- Burn ectropion Rx- release & resurface the orbicularis muscle with FTSG

53. Practice Management

- Informed consent- diagnosis, purpose of treatment/procedure, benefit, risks, complications, side effects, success rates, alternatives, consequences
- Age of informed consent is 18 years. Need one parent's consent if <18 years
- Emancipated minor criteria- marriage, having children, military service, financial independence, living apart from parents
- The ASPS defines "procedure" as "medical service that requires an incision". Cannot be donated
- Reimportation- illegal importation of drugs already approved in US from foreign country
- Malpractice- negligence in profession. Duty owed, duty breached, causation, damages
- Duty- when doctor-patient relationship is established. Doesn't have to be in person
- Photography- use same equipment on same settings for consistency, two light sources avoids flatness & shadows, blue background
- If a physician writes a prescription, he must document the encounter. State laws are variable. Federal law is limited to controlled substances
- ↑ risk of wrong-site surgery- emergency cases; unusual physical characteristics (obesity, physical deformity), time pressures, unfamiliar equipment, multiple surgeons, multiple procedures, ↑ surgeon age, experience, case volume
- MC retained foreign body- sponge. MC etiology- emergency operation, change in operation or nursing staff, >1 surgical team, ↑ BMI, ↑ blood loss, female, surgical counts
- Health Insurance Portability and Accountability Act of 1996- aka HIPAA- protects health insurance coverage when people change or lose jobs.
- Administrative simplification- national standards for electronic health care & privacy of health data
- All electronic devices with patient information or pictures must be password-protected & data properly disposed. Computer hard drives must be demagnetized or physically destroyed
- Emergency Medical Treatment & Active Labor Act- aka EMTALA- hospitals must provide care to anyone needing emergency care despite citizenship, legal status, or ability to pay
- Consolidated Omnibus Budget Reconciliation Act of 1985- aka COBRA- insurance program allows employees to continue their health insurance after leaving job
- National Health Security Strategy- plan to minimize consequences associated with significant health incidents
- Patient Protection and Affordable Care Act- reformed health insurance industry, coverage of pre-existing conditions, expands access to insurance

54. Coding

- Global period- 90 days after surgery of follow-up care without billing. Wait until global period is up before next stage of breast reconstruction. Global period for skin lesion- 1 week
- Unbundling- billing each part of a procedure
- Complicating pathology (bleeding, intertrigo, pain, pruritus) is required for Medicare to cover benign lesion excision
- Cannot bill for lesion excision & adjacent tissue transfer or arrangement
- Coding adjacent tissue transfer- area of defect + area of flap = total cm^2
- Complex closure includes debridement
- ORIF orbit floor- elevation of fracture, exploration of infraorbital nerve & orbital floor, release of entrapped orbital contents
- Radial artery free flap donor site STSG is billed separately
- Abdominal wall repair is included in TRAM
- ALT donor site closure is included
- Karapandzic technique- axial pattern musculocutaneous flap based on facial artery/vein. Billed as musculocutaneous flap
- DIEP flap code includes free TRAM, muscle-sparing TRAM, DIEP & SIEA flaps. Includes harvest, insetting, microvascular anastomosis & donor site closure
- May be added to free flap- vein graft, neurorrhaphy, nerve graft, STSG, complicated donor site closure, recipient site wound prep
- CTR 64721- incision, division of palmar aponeurosis & transverse carpal ligament, exploration of carpal tunnel, median nerve & motor branch release, epineurotomy, external neurolysis, closure, dressing, splinting & local anesthesia. Can add on internal neurolysis
- Ryan flap- not a breast reconstruction code. Code based on surface area of flap

55. Miscellaneous

- MC complication in patients undergoing combined procedures- wound healing issues (15%), seroma (10%), infection, hematoma & PE (< 5%)
- Caprini model- calculates patient risk factors for DVT
- PE- S/S- chest pain, respiratory distress, anxiety. Dx- V/Q scan, CTA, empirically start anticoagulation. Normal CXR rules out pneumonia, atelectasis, PTX. Right-sided strain on EKG is PE. Venous doppler of lower extremities. Post-op PE occurs 3-7 days after surgery, 10% fatal within 1 hour
- CHF- diastolic dysfunction due to HTN. Hypertrophied ventricular muscle can't maintain normal diastolic compliance. ↑ L ventricular filling pressures, atrial pressures, pulmonary pressure; atrial

- distension, atrial arrhythmias, V/Q mismatch, pulmonary & peripheral edema. Rx- ↓ afterload & preload
- Acute coronary syndrome- atherosclerotic plaque rupture blocks a coronary artery. S/S- chest pain, ST elevation
- Supraventricular tachycardia- normal response to adrenaline, but rule out intravascular injection. Rx- β-blockers, calcium-channel blockers, procainamide
- Virchow triad- venous stasis, vascular injury, hypercoagulability. During abdominoplasty general anesthesia & immobilization causes venous stasis. Risk of DVT is highest within 2 weeks of surgery, but remains high for 2-3 months. Risk reduction- proper patient positioning, early ambulation, knee flexion, SCDs, heparin
- HIT- platelets ↓ 30% after heparin. Rx- stop heparin. Occurs in 5% of patients on heparin, 20% of HIT patients will thrombose, 30% mortality, 30% limb loss
- Hematologic disorders (sickle cell disease)- ↑ rheologic factors cause sludging in vessel
- Factor V Leiden- resistant to inactivation by activated protein C. 3-7% of caucasians
- Garlic- ↑ bleeding due to platelet inhibitor activity
- Nicotine causes vasoconstriction; ↑ carboxyhemoglobin, platelet aggregation, blood viscosity; ↓ tissue oxygenation, collagen deposition, prostacyclin formation. All inhibit wound healing
- Post-bariatric patient's evaluation- protein-calorie intake, serum protein, vitamin & mineral status, coagulation studies, LFTs, electrolytes. Iron deficiency is MC abnormality found. Thiamine deficiency- aka Wernicke-Korsakoff encephalopathy- Rx- thiamine 100mg IV Q 8 hrs until resolution of symptoms
- Massive weight loss surgery- warm room, cover body, fluid-filled warming blankets, warm IVF, forced-air warming blankets
- Body contouring after massive weight loss- 50% complication rate. MC- wound dehiscence (early due to patient movement, late due to seroma)
- Normal body temperature during surgery ↓ infections & bleeding
- MC complications of wound vac- 1. infection 2. bleeding
- Body dysmorphic disorder- M=F, late adolescent onset, MC comorbidity- depression
- Transplant rejection
  - Hyperacute rejection- minutes to hours due to pre-formed antibodies
  - Acute humoral rejection- 3-7 days. Rx- plasmaphoresis, anti-B cell meds
  - Acute cellular rejection- 3-6 months, MC form, T-cell mediated. Rx- immunosuppressants
  - Chronic rejection- months to years, antibody & cell-mediated. Rx- immunosuppressants
- Vitamin A supplements for patients on steroids- promotes epithelialization & collagen synthesis. Rx- 20,000 IU daily
- Preoperative antibiotics given 30-59 min before incision, dosed on weight, redosed on half-life of drug or excessive blood loss

- Stop Tamoxifen 28 days before surgery
- Fluoroquinolones- arthropathy in children
- Doxycycline- discolored teeth if given < 8 years old
- Anthracycline (doxorubicin) extravasation Rx- IV dexrazoxane (or topical dimethyl sulfoxide)

56. Glossary

AD- autosomal dominant
AR- autosomal recessive
ADM- acellular dermal matrix
APL- abductor pollicis longus
BCC- basal cell carcinoma
CHF- congestive heart failure
CL/CP- cleft lip/ cleft palate
CN- cranial nerve
CRPS- chronic regional pain syndrome
CTR- carpal tunnel release
DOA- duration of action
DVT- deep venous thrombosis
ECRL- extensor carpi radialis longus
EPB- extensor pollicis brevis
F:M- female:male ratio
FCR- flexor carpi radialis
FNP- frontal nasal prominence
FTSG- full-thickness skin graft
HBO- hyperbaric oxygen
HTN- hypertension
IMF- infra-mammary fold
LNP- lateral nasal prominence
MC- most common
MNP- median nasal prominence
NAC- nipple-areola complex
N/V- nausea/vomiting
NSM- nipple-sparing mastectomy
PAD- peripheral arterial disease
PE- pulmonary embolus
PROM- passive range of motion
PT- pronator teres
PTX- pneumothorax
RCL- radial collateral ligament
RF- risk factor
Rx- treatment
S/S- signs/symptoms
SCC- squamous cell carcinoma
SE- side effects
SCM- sternocleidomastoid
SFA- superficial femoral artery
SGAP- superior gluteal artery perforator
SLNBx- sentinel lymph node biopsy
STSG- split-thickness skin graft
UA- urinalysis
UCL- ulnar collateral ligament
US- ultrasound
V/Q- ventilation/perfusion
VPI- velopharyngeal insufficiency
VRAM- vertical rectus abdominis myocutaneous
XRT- radiation

Made in the USA
Middletown, DE
04 April 2015